# Delicious Desserts When You Have Diabetes

# Delicious Desserts When You Have Diabetes

## Over 150 Recipes

Sandy Kapoor, Ph.D., R.D., F.A.D.A.

WILEY

John Wiley & Sons, Inc.

Published by John Wiley & Sons, Inc., Hoboken, New Jersey
Published simultaneously in Canada

Honey Glazed Fresh Fruit Mélange in Phyllo Tart Shells on page 146 was adapted from a recipe created by Dan Dain, John Reid, and Richard Wesley. Lemon-Flavored Cheesecake in Graham Cracker Crumb Crust on page 150, Strawberry Amaretto Glacé on page 198, and Summer-Fresh Three Berry Sauce on page 228 were adapted from recipes created by Julie Wrisley-Johnson.

For general information about our other products and services, please contact our Customer Care Department within the United States at (800) 762-2974, outside the United States at (317) 572-3993 or fax (317) 572-4002.

Wiley also publishes its books in a variety of electronic formats. Some content that appears in print may not be available in electronic books. For more information about Wiley products, visit our web site at www.wiley.com.

*Library of Congress Cataloging-in-Publication Data:*

Kapoor, Sandra.
Delicious desserts when you have diabetes : over 150 recipes / Sandy Kapoor.
p. ; cm.
ISBN 0-471-44196-1
1. Diabetes—Diet therapy—Recipes. 2. Desserts.
[DNLM: 1. Diabetes Diet—Popular Works. 2. Cookery—Popular Works. 3. Diabetes Mellitus—diet therapy—Popular Works. WK 819 K17d 2003] I. Title.
RC662 .K37 2003
641.5'6314—dc21
2002153123

Printed in the United States of America

10 9 8 7 6 5 4 3 2 1

*To the most important "boys" in my life:*
*my husband, Tarun Kapoor;*
*our six-year-old son, Tomi Kapoor;*
*my father, Curtis Kaiser;*
*and my brother, Larry Kaiser.*

# Contents

# *Preface*

Today it is estimated that about 16 million Americans (6 percent of the U.S. population) have diabetes. Until recently, it was believed that only older adults were vulnerable. Now, experts are realizing that everyone is potentially at risk—even children.

People with diabetes should eat a variety of healthy foods every day, with a focus on vegetables, fruits, whole grains, and legumes. In fact, nutritionists recommend that we eat at least five vegetables and fruits a day. These foods are nutritious, and many are excellent sources of the important vitamins A and C. They are also significant sources of folate, a B vitamin that can help reduce the risk of certain serious and common birth defects. Fruits and vegetables are high in fiber, and eating more fiber may lower blood sugar and blood cholesterol levels in people with type 2 diabetes. Vegetables and fruits also contain phytochemicals, many of which are antioxidants that help protect the body against diseases such as cancer and heart disease. Cutting back on fat, especially saturated fat, is wise since people with diabetes are at higher risk for heart disease. However, people with diabetes do not need to eat special or diet foods. And for most, it's okay to eat sugary foods *in moderation* with meals. It is the amount of carbohydrate, not the type, which is important to people with diabetes.

*Delicious Desserts When You Have Diabetes* makes eating dessert an enjoyable, healthful experience for people, whether they have diabetes or not. It contains ten chapters with a wide variety of healthy and delicious desserts. The recipes are easy-to-follow and use readily available ingredients. The measurements for the ingredients are listed by both weight and volume. To assist readers with meal planning, *Delicious Desserts When*

*You Have Diabetes* lists the yield, number of servings, and serving size for each recipe, along with nutrient content. Carbohydrate and diabetic exchanges per serving are included in the nutritional analyses.

*Delicious Desserts When You Have Diabetes* features healthy versions of many traditional favorites, including chocolate cake, banana bread, and apple pie. There is also an assortment of innovative desserts, ranging from Five-Spice Sugar-Free Cornmeal Muffins and Cakelike Dark Fudge Beanie Brownies to Blended Watermelon Cooler Flavored with Mint. Fruits and vegetables are key ingredients in many of the desserts. Many of the desserts are also prepared with whole grains or their products. In addition to being richer in vitamins, minerals, and fiber, these desserts are low in cholesterol, total and saturated fat, and contain less sugar and salt than their traditional counterparts. But most important, the desserts in *Delicious Desserts When You Have Diabetes* are unbelievably delicious.

# Acknowledgments

The recipes in *Delicious Desserts When You Have Diabetes* are the result of five years of development, testing, and tasting—and retesting and tasting—along with ongoing nutritional analyses and calculation of diabetic exchanges. There is only one word for the hard work of the many talented, creative, and diligent California State Polytechnic University, Pomona, Collins School of Hospitality Management student research assistants who have participated in this project: *awesome*. I thank them all for their contributions.

I also thank my husband, Tarun Kapoor, a person with both diabetes and heart disease; our six-year-old-son, Tomi Kapoor; and my friends Mayra Brown, Dan Brown, Gary Hamilton, and Ardel Nelson for their valued suggestions and advice throughout the many stages in the development of these recipes. In order to receive the approval of this diverse group's very critical and sensitive palates, these desserts had to taste *good*.

I am grateful to my mother, Harriette Kaiser, for inspiring many of these recipes and teaching me how to cook.

I am most appreciative to California State Polytechnic University for its support in helping me to bring this project to fruition.

Finally, thank you to my editor, Elizabeth Zack, and copy editor, Miriam Sarzin.

# *Introduction*

The best part of a meal for many people is dessert. *Delicious Desserts When You Have Diabetes* provides recipes for people who love dessert but want to eat healthily, too. These desserts are not difficult to make, but do require having the right ingredients, measuring accurately, and carefully following the directions. Here are some helpful tips.

## ABOUT THE INGREDIENTS

If nutrient analyses are to be accurate, you must carefully measure the ingredients as specified in the recipes and make sure to divide the recipes into the designated number of servings. This is important to do when you are cooking for people with diabetes.

## FORM OF INGREDIENTS

The way ingredients are measured, such as firmly packed brown sugar or unsifted powdered sugar, is described in the ingredient list. Any ingredient preparation required before or after measuring, such as mincing herbs; chopping nuts; thawing fruit juice concentrate; or peeling, coring, slicing, dicing, or puréeing fruits and vegetables, is noted in the ingredient list.

For example, a recipe in which peaches need to be peeled and thinly sliced *before* measuring lists the peaches in the following manner:

| | WEIGHT | MEASURE |
|---|---|---|
| Peeled and thinly sliced fresh ripe peaches | 26 oz | 4½ c (1⅛ qt) |

But a recipe calling for whole peaches to be peeled and thinly sliced *after* measuring lists the peaches as follows:

| | WEIGHT | MEASURE |
|---|---|---|
| Fresh ripe peaches, peeled and thinly sliced | 16 oz as purchased | 3 medium/ 2 large |

For the best results, measure the ingredients as listed in the recipes.

## WEIGHING AND MEASURING INGREDIENTS

Both weights (ounces and pounds) and volumes (quarts, pints, cups, table-spoons, teaspoons) are listed for most solid ingredients unless the amount is less than one ounce. Weighing these ingredients is the preferred and most accurate method of measuring and was the method used to develop and test these recipes. Weights of ingredients should be measured with a scale, preferably an electronic scale.

Either shell or liquid eggs can be used in the recipes. Shell eggs should be large.

Observe these rules when measuring the following ingredients.

- Measure flour by gently spooning it into a dry measuring cup. Don't pack it down. Then level it off by sliding a table knife over the rim of the cup and letting the excess fall back into the bag.
- If brown sugar is called for, the recipe will specify how the brown sugar should be packed in the cup (firmly packed, lightly packed, unpacked). Pack the cup according to recipe specifications before leveling it off.
- For ingredients such as flaked coconut and chopped nuts, fill the cup and *then* level it off with your fingers.
- When measuring small amounts of ingredients, begin with clean and dry measuring spoons. Then, scoop ingredients to overflowing, and level them off with a table knife.
- Measure liquid ingredients with a glass measuring cup for easier reading. Place the liquid measuring cup on a level surface and bend

down to read it at eye level while pouring to the correct mark. A 2-cup (pint) measure is standard and a 4-cup (quart) measure is helpful to have on hand.

- In a few recipes, a *scant* amount (for example, scant 1 tablespoon gelatin, scant 1 cup flour) of an ingredient is called for. Use just a little less than the measure listed. For example, for 1 scant tablespoon, use 2½ teaspoons (1 tablespoon minus ½ teaspoon) and for 1 scant cup, use ¾ cup + 3 tablespoons (1 cup minus 1 tablespoon).
- When a recipe calls for a *pinch* of an ingredient (for example, a pinch of cloves, pinch of ground ginger), add about ¹⁄₁₆ teaspoon, or as much as can be taken between your thumb and forefinger.

## ABBREVIATIONS

The following abbreviations are used.

| | | | |
|---|---|---|---|
| c | cup | pt | pint |
| F | Fahrenheit | poly | polyunsaturated |
| g | gram | qt | quart |
| lb | pound | sat | saturated |
| mg | milligram | tbsp | tablespoon |
| mono | monounsaturated | tsp | teaspoon |
| oz | ounce | | |

## PREPARATION OF EQUIPMENT

Small, medium, and large bowls, saucepans, and storage containers are called for in recipes.

- Small—1 quart (4 cups)
- Medium—2 quarts (8 cups)
- Large—3 quarts (12 cups)

An ice cream freezer is preferred for making the frozen yogurts, sherbets, ice creams, sorbets, and other frozen desserts. For those without an ice cream freezer, directions are also provided for preparing the desserts by freezing in shallow, nonreactive metal pans and beating with an electric mixer or blending in a food processor or blender. However, frozen desserts prepared in an ice cream freezer will have a smoother texture.

## FRUITS AND VEGETABLES

Most recipe books for desserts begin with a selection of cakes followed by bars and cookies. Typically, a brief list of fruit desserts is included near the end. Because fruit desserts are so delicious to eat and so good for us, *Delicious Desserts When You Have Diabetes* begins with a chapter of fresh fruit desserts, followed by a chapter of cooked fruit desserts to encourage you to eat more fruit desserts. Remember that fruits are nutritious, full of vitamins and minerals. Their fiber and phytochemical content can help control blood sugar and protect against cancer and heart disease.

Fruits and vegetables are also added to enhance the taste, texture, and nutritional profile of the desserts in every chapter. Fruits and vegetables are blended into many of the cakes, cookies, bars, and quick breads. Gelatins, ice creams and other frozen desserts, and smoothies are prepared with a variety of fruits and vegetables. Recipes for pies, cheesecakes, and sauces featuring fruits and vegetables are offered.

Fresh fruit is used in recipes unless otherwise specified. Make sure to always wash (and dry) fresh fruits and vegetables before using. When recipes call for frozen fruit, thaw and drain it before measuring it unless told otherwise.

Several recipes call for baking apples. Some good choices of uniform-size apples that stay firm and flavorful when baked are Cortland, Northern Spy, Rome Beauty, Winesap, and York Imperial apples.

Many other recipes call for tart apples. Good choices include Cortland, Gravenstein, Granny Smith, Grimes Golden, Jonathan, McIntosh, Newton Pippin, Northern Spy, Rhode Island Greening, Stayman, Winesap, and York Imperial.

## FATS AND OILS

Heart disease is the leading complication and cause of death in people with diabetes. For this reason, cutting back on fat, especially saturated fat, is key. Several techniques are employed to minimize the total and saturated fat and cholesterol in these dessert recipes.

For starters, lard, shortening, and butter are not used in the recipes. Most of the desserts are made with no added fat, or small amounts of olive oil, rich in monounsaturated fat or margarine, rich in polyunsaturated fat. Baking pans and trays are sprayed with butter-flavored vegetable cooking oil rather than coating them with the traditional shortening, butter, or margarine.

Traditionally, most baked goods are high in fat. A variety of ingredients replace the fat in these baked goods. They include fat-free yogurt, fat-free sour cream, and fruit and vegetable purées including apricot, banana, dried plum (prune), kidney bean, pumpkin and sweet potato purées, and applesauce.

Prune purée is particularly effective as a fat substitute in baked goods. It replaces the fat in many of the cakes, cookies, bars, and quick breads. Prune purée's success is attributed to it being rich in three ingredients: pectin, sorbitol, and malic acid. Pectin is a type of dietary fiber that entraps air just as effectively as shortening to produce good texture in baked goods. Sorbitol is a mildly sweet alcohol sugar that keeps baked goods soft and moist, providing them with the mouthfeel typically associated with their higher-fat counterparts. Finally, the malic acid in prunes acts as a flavor enhancer as well as a natural preservative.

To make prune purée, combine 8 ounces (1⅓ cups) pitted prunes and 6 tablespoons of hot water in a food processor or blender. Pulse on and off until the prunes are finely chopped and nearly smooth. If you prefer not to make your own, prune baby food works well, too.

Frostings and toppings for baked goods are also usually rich in butter, shortening, or margarine, and contain other ingredients high in fat, saturated fat, and cholesterol, such as cream cheese, egg yolks, whole milk, and cream. The frostings and toppings in *Delicious Desserts When You Have Diabetes* are made without butter, shortening, margarine, or other added fat.

Pastries are traditionally made with lard, shortening, butter, and more recently, margarine. To minimize the fat in these pastries, pies are made with only one reduced-fat crust or topped with reduced-fat pastry cutouts, lower-fat crumb toppings, or a fat- and cholesterol-free egg white meringue. In other pies, high-fat and high-cholesterol crusts are replaced with a reduced-fat crisp egg white meringue shell, phyllo shell, or cereal crust.

## EGGS

To reduce the total and saturated fat and cholesterol in the desserts, few recipes require egg yolks. Many of the baked goods, including cakes, cookies, and quick breads, contain no egg yolks, or just one yolk per recipe. Egg whites, baking soda, or baking powder serve as leavening agents in many of the baked goods, and fruit and vegetable purées are used to enhance their taste, texture, and mouthfeel.

Desserts such as pastry fillings and sauces are thickened and enriched with starches, vegetable and fruit purées, and lower-fat dairy products (such as fat-free cream cheese and fat-free sweetened condensed milk) instead of whole eggs or egg yolks. One or two egg yolks might be added per recipe.

Many of the recipes call for egg whites. Liquid egg whites eliminate the tedious process of separating egg yolks from their whites as well as the hassle of leftover yolks. Products containing 100 percent pasteurized liquid egg whites with no preservatives or additives are readily available in the refrigerated section of most major supermarkets and specialty food stores.

In a few of the recipes (for example, Blackberry Snow Tart, Lime Chiffon Angel Pie, and Pumpkin Chiffon Pie Dashed with Orange) the eggs are not cooked. Any time a recipe calls for raw eggs, salmonella infection is a concern. To be worry-free when making recipes in which eggs are not completely cooked, choose pasteurized eggs. While pasteurized liquid eggs have been around for some time, pasteurization of shell eggs is a relatively new thing. Davidson's Pasteurized Shell Eggs are available in many supermarkets, but if you cannot find them in your area, visit www.davidsonseggs.com for more information.

Egg substitutes are intentionally not used in the recipes. While there is a whole range of liquid products available that have been formulated with less total fat, saturated fat, cholesterol, and/or calories to substitute for real eggs, they contain varying levels of fat and cholesterol. Most are made from egg whites and other ingredients (oil, milk products, artificial color, emulsifiers, antioxidants, vitamins, and minerals) designed to simulate the yolk's color, flavor, texture, nutritional value, and mouthfeel. They are generally more expensive than fresh egg whites, often contain additives, and usually are higher in calories.

## DAIRY PRODUCTS

Dairy products—including cream, half-and-half, whole milk, ice cream, whole milk yogurt, whole milk frozen yogurt, sour cream, cream cheese, evaporated whole milk, and sweetened condensed whole milk—are all high in total and saturated fat and cholesterol. They are replaced with a variety of lower-fat and lower-cholesterol dairy products in these recipes. They include fat-free half-and-half, fat-free or low-fat milk, low-fat buttermilk, low-fat or reduced-fat ice cream, fat-free yogurt, fat-free or low-fat frozen yogurt, fat-free cream cheese, fat-free evaporated milk, and fat-free sweetened condensed milk.

## WHOLE GRAINS

The government recommends that we make at least three of our daily grain-based foods whole grain. The fiber in whole grains helps to reduce blood levels of "bad" LDL cholesterol and maintain proper bowel function, heading off constipation as well as more serious conditions, such as diverticulitis. Eating more fiber can be beneficial for both preventing and treating diabetes, too. Whole grain foods also contribute vitamin E, selenium, and zinc—nutrients that are not added back when refined grains are enriched.

## SWEETENING AGENTS

Many of the desserts are prepared with whole grains and their products such as bran flakes, granola, oats, oat bran, stone ground yellow cornmeal, white whole wheat flour, whole wheat English muffins, and whole wheat flour.

Only natural sugars are used in the recipes—no artificial sweeteners. For most people with diabetes, it's okay to eat sugar in moderation. Just like starch, sugar is a carbohydrate, and both sugar and starch can raise blood glucose levels. It's the *amount* of carbohydrate, not the source, that matters.

Many of the desserts are sweetened with fruit—fresh, frozen, canned, or dried—and fruit purées, spreads, juices, or juice concentrates, alone or in combination with other sweetening agents. While molasses, maple syrup, honey, and brown sugar are not significantly more nutritious than granulated sugar, they serve as sweetening agents in many of these desserts because of their rich or light and creamy flavor, full body, or ability to hold moisture or yield a smooth texture. Additionally, honey has a milder effect on blood sugar than other carbohydrates because the sugar it contains is one-third to one-half fructose, which is absorbed without triggering insulin.

Another method employed to reduce the sugar in these desserts is to enhance their sweetness with a sprinkle of sweet spice or a splash of flavor extract. It is also recommended that sweet frostings or syrups on desserts such as cakes, bars, soft cookies, and pancakes be eliminated, reduced, or replaced with a fruit sauce or spread, sliced fruit, or a scoop of reduced-sugar and reduced-fat frozen yogurt or ice cream. To further maximize their sweet flavor, serve desserts, including baked goods, cooked fruit desserts, puddings, custards, and flans warm or at room temperature rather than chilled. Even frozen desserts will taste sweeter if served slightly softened rather than frozen hard.

## SALT

Salt is a concern of some diners. It is either eliminated or reduced in most of these recipes. Instead, flavor is heightened with a splash of citrus juice, vinegar, a flavor extract, wine, or liqueur.

In some of the desserts, the flavor is enhanced with a sprinkle of freshly grated citrus zest, grated fresh ginger, minced fresh mint, a mixture of aromatic spices, or a few seeds toasted without fat. Fruits, too, are loaded with taste. Diced and sliced fresh, frozen, and canned and dried fruits and their purées, spreads, juices, and juice concentrates, as well as vegetables and their purées, are blended into many of the desserts to enrich their flavor. In some cases, desserts are given a rich and hearty flavor by replacing a refined grain, flour, or bread with a whole grain product.

## OTHER INGREDIENTS

A variety of other ingredients and cooking techniques are employed to maximize the delicious taste and nutritional value of these recipes. This is a brief list:

- Green or black tea as a primary ingredient in beverages
- Soy foods (soy flour, tofu, soy milk, or soy nut butter) featured in pies, quick breads, cooked fruits, and beverages
- Cocoa powder substituted for chocolate
- Coconut and nuts replaced with dried fruit bits or minimized by toasting (to heighten flavor) or by combining less with an extract

# Computing Nutrients
## in Recipes

### NUTRIENT ANALYSIS

Each recipe has been analyzed for calories, grams of fat, saturated fat, monounsaturated fat, polyunsaturated fat, protein, carbohydrates, alcohol, and dietary fiber, and milligrams of cholesterol, sodium, iron, and calcium per serving. The percentage of calories from fat, carbohydrates, protein, and alcohol per serving are also listed. In a few situations, information was not available about the nutritional value of key ingredients in recipes; this is reflected in the analysis with a dash before the nutrient.

The calorie and nutrient breakdown for each recipe was derived from computer analysis (The Food Processor; Version 7.8; ESHA Research, P.O. Box 13028, Salem, OR 97309). The program gathered its information primarily from the U.S. Department of Agriculture.

The calorie and nutrient values are as accurate as possible. The following assumptions were made:

- Dishes are prepared with only the ingredients listed. In the event more or less or another form of ingredient is used or an ingredient is eliminated from or added to a recipe, the nutrient analysis does not reflect these adjustments.
- Calories and nutrient values listed are per serving.
- The serving size is designed to reflect the way health-conscious people eat, common portion size, or in some cases, by dividing the product yield in the manner that seemed most reasonable for the recipe.

- Since a percentage of alcohol calories evaporate when heated, this reduction is estimated in the nutrient analysis.
- Nutrient analysis is calculated for natural flavor extracts (such as almond, lemon, and anise) with alcohol except vanilla. Because most cooks use imitation vanilla extract without alcohol, the nutrient analysis reflects this.
- Garnishes and other optional ingredients, toppings, and companion foods are not included in the nutrient analysis.
- When a dash denotes an ingredient's amount, for example, vegetable oil cooking spray, it is not included in the nutrient analysis.
- When more than one ingredient is listed as an option, the nutrient analysis is conducted on the first ingredient listed.
- Energy is rounded off to the nearest calorie and the nutrients to the nearest tenth per serving.

## DIABETIC EXCHANGES

Diabetic exchanges are listed per serving for each recipe. *Please note:* When calculating exchange values for the recipes per serving, the best match possible was made between the actual energy and nutrient values per serving and the exchange values.

- Actual carbohydrate values are within ± 5 grams of the exchange value.
- Protein values are within ± 3 grams of the exchange value.
- Fat values are within ± 2 grams of the exchange value.
- Energy values are within ± 20 calories.

*Please also be aware:*

- Exchanges of ¼ or ⅓, and meat exchanges of ½ are not included.
- A free food contains less than 20 calories or less than 5 grams carbohydrate per serving.
- There are five choices (starch, fruit, milk, other carbohydrates, or vegetables) in the carbohydrate group. The specific type of carbohydrate is identified in these recipes.

# Fresh Fruit Desserts

Banana Boats Filled with Sliced Mixed Fruit

Cantaloupe Balls Sprinkled with Blueberries

Creamy Fruit Salad with Marshmallows

Fresh Fruit and Strawberry Cream Cheese Tortilla Pizza

Fresh Fruit Layered with Shredded Coconut

Fresh Fruit Medley Sprinkled with Poppy Seeds

Fresh Fruit, Peach Yogurt, and Granola Parfaits

Honeydew Balls Laced with Pernod

Honey-Sweetened Medley of Fresh Fruit

Layered Raspberries, Bing Cherries, and Oranges

Minted Melon Balls Marinated in Fruit Juice Syrup

Navel Oranges and Kiwis Sprinkled with Berries in
Rose-Scented Syrup

Orange Sections in Raspberry Syrup Splashed with Chambord

Papaya Banana Sauce Sweetened with Fruit Juice

Pineapple Wedges Decorated with Melon Balls

Sliced Strawberries Macerated in Port

Summer Fruit Layered with Vanilla Amaretto Custard Sauce

Watermelon and Raspberries in Light Raspberry Glaze

# Banana Boats Filled with Sliced Mixed Fruit

*If you aren't a believer of the claim "we eat with our eyes," watch diners' reactions when this simple mixture of sliced fruit is presented in a banana shell. It offers an impressive dessert and at the same time, it is easy to make.*

YIELD: 4 banana boats                    SERVING SIZE: 1 banana boat

|  | WEIGHT | MEASURE |
|---|---|---|
| Ripe bananas | 1½ lb as purchased | 4 medium |
| Mandarin oranges canned in light syrup, drained | 11-oz can | 1 c drained |
| Hulled and sliced fresh ripe strawberries | 6 oz | 1 c |
| Orange juice |  | ¼ c |
| Kiwis, peeled and sliced | 6 oz as purchased | 2 medium |

With a small pointed knife, cut a strip of peel about 1 inch wide from each banana. Begin cutting strip at inside tip of each banana and continue cutting strip until about ½ inch from stem, leaving strip and stem attached. Remove banana from peel. Roll strip of peel over stem and secure with a wooden or plastic pick. Top pick with mandarin orange and strawberry slice.

Slice bananas obliquely or on a diagonal. Place in a large bowl. Pour orange juice over bananas to prevent browning. Add remaining fruit and mix gently. Spoon fruit mixture attractively into banana shells. Serve immediately.

---

### NUTRITIONAL FACTS

| | | |
|---|---|---|
| Calories: 172 (5% from fat) | Carbohydrate: 43 g and 90% | Sodium: 4.3 mg |
| Fat: 1 g (.3 g sat, .1 g mono, .3 g poly) | Fiber: 6.3 g | Calcium: 32.4 mg |
| Protein: 2.3 g and 5% | Cholesterol: 0 mg | Diabetic Exchanges: 3 Fruits |
| | Iron: .8 mg | |

# Cantaloupe Balls Sprinkled with Blueberries

Nutrition Action Healthletter *rates cantaloupe as one of the ten super-foods you should eat. It's no wonder. A quarter of a melon supplies almost as much vitamins A and C as most people need in an entire day.*

*While there is no sure way to determine the quality of a cantaloupe from the outside, there are some fairly reliable indicators to use when purchasing. Look for a slightly oval melon with a diameter of five inches or more and a slight golden, or, at worst, light greenish gray (not dull, dark green) background color under the netting. Signs of sweetness are pronounced netting and a few tiny cracks near the stem end. If you shake the melon and hear a slight rattling of the seeds, it may be extra sweet, but more than likely it's overripe and slightly sour.*

*In this simple yet attractive dessert, balls of the musky-sweet but slightly tart melon are gently tossed with crunchy textured, sweet and mild blueberries and enhanced with fruit juices and a sprinkle of grated fresh gingerroot.*

YIELD: 4½ c (1⅛ qt) fruit　　　　　　　　　　SERVINGS: 9
SERVING SIZE: ½ c fruit

| | WEIGHT | MEASURE |
|---|---|---|
| Thawed white grape juice concentrate, undiluted | | 3 tbsp |
| Fresh lime juice | | 2 tbsp |
| Finely grated lime zest | | 2 tsp |
| Peeled and minced gingerroot | | 1 tsp |
| ½-inch cantaloupe balls (1 medium—3¼ lb— melon) | 22 oz | 4 c (1 qt) |
| Fresh ripe blueberries | 5 oz | 1 c |

Combine grape juice concentrate, lime juice and zest, and gingerroot in a small bowl. Mix until blended.

Combine cantaloupe and blueberries in a medium bowl. Pour juice mixture over fruit. Toss gently to coat. Spoon into 9 stemmed glasses or small dessert dishes and serve.

---

### NUTRITIONAL FACTS

Calories: 45 (5% from fat)

Fat: .3 g (.1 g sat, 0 g mono, .1 g poly)

Protein: .8 g and 6%

Carbohydrate: 11.1 g and 89%

Fiber: 1.1 g

Cholesterol: 0 mg

Iron: .2 mg

Sodium: 7.7 mg

Calcium: 10.4 mg

Diabetic Exchanges: 1 Fruit

---

# Creamy Fruit Salad with Marshmallows

*This fruit salad is like a sweet gelatin and can be served as either a salad or a dessert. A few simple steps reduce the fat, sugar, and calories and enhance the flavor and eye appeal of the traditional easy-to-make favorite. Begin with fruit packed in its own juice or light rather than heavy syrup. Combine the fruits with pastel colored marshmallows and toast the flaked sweetened coconut. (To toast coconut and pecans, cook separately over medium heat in a dry nonstick skillet, stirring constantly until coconut is golden brown and nuts are just beginning to become fragrant.) Finally, replace the sour cream with fat-free sour cream and sweeten and flavor with fruit spread rather than heavy syrup.*

YIELD: 3 c (1½ pt) fruit salad  
SERVING SIZE: ½ c fruit salad

SERVINGS: 6

| | WEIGHT | MEASURE |
|---|---|---|
| Fat-free sour cream | 8-oz carton | scant 1 c |
| 100%-fruit peach spread | | 1 tbsp |
| Pineapple chunks canned in juice, drained | 8¼-oz can | ¾ c drained |
| Mandarin oranges canned in light syrup, drained | 11-oz can | 1 c drained |
| Miniature colored marshmallows | 2 oz | 1 c |
| Flaked sweetened coconut, toasted without fat | 3 oz | 1 c |
| Pecans, chopped and toasted without fat | | 2 tbsp |

Combine sour cream and peach spread in a medium bowl. Mix until blended. Add pineapple, mandarin oranges, marshmallows, and coconut. Mix until coated. Cover and refrigerate until chilled. Spoon into 6 dessert dishes. Sprinkle with chopped pecans and serve.

---

### NUTRITIONAL FACTS

Calories: 189 (29% from fat)
Fat: 6.5 g (4.2 g sat, 1.2 g
   mono, .6 g poly)
Protein: 3.8 g and 8%

Carbohydrate: 31 g and
   63%
Fiber: 1.9 g
Cholesterol: 0 mg
Iron: .5 mg
Sodium: 79.3 mg

Calcium 83.5 mg
Diabetic Exchanges: 1
   Other Carbohydrate;
   ½ Fruit; ½ Low-Fat
   Milk; 1 Fat

---

# Fresh Fruit and Strawberry Cream Cheese Tortilla Pizza

*This easy-to-make and colorful pizza is a fun conclusion to a meal. Oven-crisped 98% fat-free tortillas are spread with pink strawberry-flavored fat-free cream cheese, decorated with sliced fruit, and sprinkled with toasted flaked sweetened coconut.*

YIELD: two 8-inch fruit pizzas          SERVINGS: 4
SERVING SIZE: ½ fruit pizza

| | WEIGHT | MEASURE |
|---|---|---|
| 98% fat-free 8-inch flour tortillas | | 2 |
| Butter-flavored vegetable oil cooking spray | — | — |
| Flaked sweetened coconut, toasted without fat | | 2 tbsp |
| Block-style fat-free cream cheese | 4 oz | ½ c |
| 100%-fruit strawberry spread | 3 oz | ¼ c |
| Vanilla extract | | ½ tsp |
| Fresh ripe strawberries, hulled and sliced | 6 oz as purchased | 6 large (1 c sliced) |
| Halved seedless green grapes | 6 oz | 1 c |
| Fresh ripe blueberries | 3 oz | ½ c |

Preheat oven to 400 degrees F.

Place tortillas on a baking sheet. Lightly coat top with cooking spray. Bake until crisp, or about 5 minutes. Cool.

Toast coconut by cooking over medium heat in a dry nonstick skillet, stirring constantly until golden brown. Set aside.

Combine cream cheese, strawberry spread, and vanilla in a small bowl. Beat until well mixed and light and airy. Spread half the cream cheese mixture on each tortilla.

Arrange half each of strawberries, grapes, and blueberries decoratively on each tortilla. Sprinkle half the toasted coconut over each. Cut into fourths and serve. Store refrigerated.

---

### NUTRITIONAL FACTS

| | | |
|---|---|---|
| Calories: 193 (10% from fat) | Carbohydrate: 37.5 g and 76% | Sodium: 331.2 mg |
| Fat: 2.1 g (1.3 g sat, .2 g mono, .2 g poly) | Fiber: 3 g | Calcium: 84.4 mg |
| Protein: 7 g and 14% | Cholesterol: 2.3 mg | Diabetic Exchanges: 1 Starch; 1 Fruit; ½ Low-Fat Milk |
| | Iron: 1.1 mg | |

# Fresh Fruit Layered with Shredded Coconut

*A dish of fresh, ripe, sweet fruit makes a nice ending to almost any meal. For a special touch, offer the fruit in stemmed glasses layered with grated fresh coconut.*

*To open a fresh coconut, pierce one or two of the three dark-colored eyes at the top of the nut with a screwdriver or ice pick. Drain out the liquid inside (reserve it for another use or drink it). Place the coconut on a baking pan in a 350-degree F oven until the shell begins to crack, or about 15 minutes. Cool briefly. Place on a sturdy surface. Using a hammer or mallet, hit the coconut hard along the crack. The nut should break into pieces. Remove the white coconut flesh from the shell with a screwdriver or knife with a rounded end. Peel away the brown skin with a small sharp knife or vegetable peeler. Coconuts yield about half their original weight after hulling and draining. A medium-size coconut will yield about three or four cups of grated coconut. An unopened coconut will keep in the refrigerator crisper for up to one month. Once opened, cover the coconut meat tightly and refrigerate for up to four days or freeze for up to six months. Grate a few chunks at a time with a hand grater, food processor, or blender.*

YIELD: 6 c (1½ qt) fruit　　　　　　　　　　　SERVINGS: 12
SERVING SIZE: ½ c fruit

| | WEIGHT | MEASURE |
|---|---|---|
| Peeled and sliced kiwis (about 3 large) | 6 oz | 1 c |
| Peeled and cubed mango (about 1 medium) | 6 oz | 1 c |
| Peeled and sliced bananas (about 2 small) | 6 oz | 1 c |
| Peeled and cubed papaya (about 1 very small) | 6 oz | 1 c |
| Hulled and sliced fresh ripe strawberries | 12 oz | 2 c (1 pt) |
| Unsweetened grated fresh coconut or | | |
| unsweetened or sweetened flaked coconut | 1½ oz | ½ c |
| Fresh orange juice | | ¼ c + 2 tbsp |
| Orange-flavored liqueur | | 2 tbsp |

Layer the fruit in a medium glass serving bowl or 12 stemmed glasses, sprinkling coconut between layers. Sprinkle coconut on top. Drizzle orange juice and orange-flavored liqueur over and serve.

## NUTRITIONAL FACTS

Calories: 82 (16% from fat)

Fat: 1.6 g (1.1 g sat, .1 g mono, .2 g poly)

Protein: 1 g and 4%

Carbohydrate: 16.7 g and 75%

Alcohol: .6 g and 5%

Fiber: 2.8 g

Cholesterol: 0 mg

Iron: .4 mg

Sodium: 3.3 mg

Calcium: 17.6 mg

Diabetic Exchanges: 1 Fruit; ½ Fat

# Fresh Fruit Medley Sprinkled with Poppy Seeds

*Before I became more experienced in the kitchen, I automatically avoided any recipe that called for citrus fruit sections. When I finally tested my skill on a few oranges, I was amazed at how easy the process is.*

*If you are new to the kitchen, follow these steps to section the oranges and grapefruit in this recipe: Cut a slice from the top and bottom of the fruit with a serrated knife to expose its flesh. Then stand the fruit on end and remove the peel and all the white membrane by cutting deeply with downward strokes. Holding the fruit in one hand over a container (large enough to hold the fruit and collect the juice), cut out each fruit section to free it from its membrane. (It should be free of its membrane and white pith.) Store the sections in the container with the juice until you are ready to use them.*

YIELD: 5 c (1¼ qt) fruit

SERVING SIZE: ½ c fruit

SERVINGS: 10

| | WEIGHT | MEASURE |
|---|---|---|
| Fresh orange juice | | ¼ c + 2 tbsp |
| Thawed white grape juice concentrate, undiluted | | 2 tbsp |
| Poppy seeds | | 1 tbsp |
| Almond extract | | ¼ tsp |
| Oranges, sectioned with juice | 1 lb as purchased | 3 medium |
| Pink-fleshed grapefruit, sectioned with juice | 15 oz as purchased | 1 medium |
| Halved seedless green grapes | 6 oz | 1 c |
| Ripe banana | 6 oz as purchased | 1 medium |
| Hulled and sliced fresh ripe strawberries | 6 oz | 1 c |

Combine orange juice, grape juice concentrate, poppy seeds, and almond extract in a small bowl. Mix well.

Combine citrus fruits and grapes in a storage container. Pour juice mixture over and mix gently. Chill.

Just before serving, peel and slice banana into ½-inch rounds. Add bananas and strawberries to chilled fruit. Mix gently. Arrange fruit in 10 chilled stemmed glasses or dessert dishes. Garnish with mint sprigs, if desired, and serve.

```
NUTRITIONAL FACTS
```

| | | |
|---|---|---|
| Calories: 74 (8% from fat) | Carbohydrate: 19.9 g and 86% | Iron: .7 mg |
| Fat: .8 g (.1 g sat, .1 g mono, .4 g poly) | Alcohol: .1 g and 1% | Sodium: 2.1 mg |
| Protein: 1.4 g and 6% | Fiber: 3.6 g | Calcium: 55 mg |
| | Cholesterol: 0 mg | Diabetic Exchanges: 1½ Fruits |

# Fresh Fruit, Peach Yogurt, and Granola Parfaits

*A mixture of brightly colored ripe sweet berries is layered in parfait glasses with fat- and sugar-free peach-flavored yogurt and granola with no added fat. This easy-to-make, good-looking, and good-tasting dessert packs lots of nutrition.*

YIELD: 6 c (1½ qt) parfaits         SERVINGS: 6
SERVING SIZE: 1 c parfait

| | WEIGHT | MEASURE |
|---|---|---|
| Mixed fresh, ripe berries (blackberries, blueberries, gooseberries, raspberries, red currants, strawberries) | 1¼ lb as purchased | 4 c (1 qt) |
| Fat-free plain yogurt | 13 oz | 1½ c |
| 100%-fruit peach spread | 4 oz | ¼ c + 2 tbsp |
| Granola with no added fat | 7½ oz | 2 c (1 pt) |

Hull berries or remove blossom and/or stem ends as needed. Cut into ½-inch dice if large.

Combine yogurt and peach spread in a small bowl. Beat until well blended. Alternate 3 or 4 layers of fruit, yogurt, and granola in 6 parfait or pilsner glasses and serve.

---

### NUTRITIONAL FACTS

Calories: 257 (9% from fat)
Fat: 2.9 g (.5 g sat, .1 g mono, .2 g poly)
Protein: 13 g and 18%

Carbohydrate: 53.1 g and 73%
Fiber: 7.3 g
Cholesterol: 1.2 mg
Iron: 1.3 mg
Sodium: 60.3 mg

Calcium: 160.7 mg
Diabetic Exchanges: 1 Starch; ½ Other Carbohydrate; 1 Fruit; ½ Skim Milk; ½ Low-Fat Milk

# Honeydew Balls
# Laced with Pernod

*This recipe calls for the licorice-flavored liqueur, Pernod, France's modern-day form of absinthe. Absinthe was banned throughout much of the world in 1915 when stories spread that its ingestion could cause complications such as convulsions, mania, hallucinations, loss of hearing and sight, and in large doses, coma and even death.*

*To create Pernod, absinthe's toxic main ingredient, wormwood, was replaced with anise and its alcohol content lowered from 136 to 86 proof. When not available, replace Pernod in this and other recipes with another anise-based spirit.*

YIELD: 6 c (1½ qt) honeydew balls          SERVINGS: 12
SERVING SIZE: ½ c honeydew balls

|  | WEIGHT | MEASURE |
|---|---|---|
| Ripe honeydew melon | 5 lb as purchased | 1 medium |
| Pernod or other anise-based spirit |  | 3 tbsp |
| Fresh lime juice |  | 2 tbsp |
| Finely grated lime zest |  | 2 tsp |

Cut melon in half and remove seeds. Cut round melon balls by pressing large end of a melon baller deep into flesh, twisting, and removing. Place balls in a storage container.

Combine Pernod and lime juice in a small bowl. Mix until blended. Pour over melon balls, turning to coat. Cover and refrigerate. Marinate fruit, turning occasionally, until honeydew is permeated with anise flavor, or about 3 hours.

Spoon into 12 chilled stemmed glasses or dessert dishes. Sprinkle with lime zest and serve.

---

NUTRITIONAL FACTS

Calories: 45 (2% from fat)   Alcohol: .9 g and 13%   Sodium: 9.1 mg
Fat: .1 g                    Fiber: .6 g             Calcium: 6.1 mg
Protein: .4 g and 3%         Cholesterol: 0 mg       Diabetic Exchanges:
Carbohydrate: 10 g and       Iron: .1 mg                 ½ Fruit
    82%

# Honey-Sweetened Medley of Fresh Fruit

*This fruit medley is as good to eat as it is to look at. A brightly colored assortment of attractively cut fruit is coated with a light honey-sweetened sauce and finished with a pinch of lime zest and ground ginger. Offer the vitamin-rich mixture for breakfast along with a whole grain English muffin and low-fat yogurt, or serve it as a healthy midday snack or an enjoyable conclusion to lunch or dinner. It's sure to bring smiles.*

YIELD: 4 c (1qt) fruit                                      SERVINGS: 8
SERVING SIZE: ½ c fruit

|  | WEIGHT | MEASURE |
| --- | --- | --- |
| ½-inch cantaloupe balls or cubes | 6 oz | 1 c |
| Peeled, cored and cubed pineapple | 6 oz | 1 c |
| Hulled and halved fresh ripe strawberries | 6 oz | 1 c |
| Seedless green grapes | 5 oz | 1 c |
| Fresh orange juice |  | ¼ c |
| Honey |  | 2 tbsp |
| Finely grated lime zest |  | ½ tsp |
| Fresh lime juice |  | 2 tsp |
| Ground ginger |  | ⅛ tsp |
| Fresh ripe blueberries | 4 oz | ¾ c |

Combine cantaloupe, pineapple, strawberries, and grapes in a medium storage container.

Combine orange juice, honey, lime zest and juice, and ginger in a small bowl. Mix until blended. Pour over fruit mixture. Cover and refrigerate until chilled.

Toss gently to mix. Spoon into 8 chilled dessert dishes or stemmed glasses. Sprinkle with blueberries and serve.

```
┌─────────────────────────────────────────────────────────────────┐
│                      NUTRITIONAL FACTS                            │
│                                                                   │
│ Calories: 65 (5% from fat)   Carbohydrate: 16.3 g and   Sodium: 3.9 mg      │
│ Fat: .4 g (.1 g sat, 0 g        91%                     Calcium: 10.9 mg    │
│    mono, .2 g poly)          Fiber: 1.5 g               Diabetic Exchanges: 1│
│ Protein: .7 g and 4%         Cholesterol: 0 mg             Fruit            │
│                              Iron: .3 mg                          │
└─────────────────────────────────────────────────────────────────┘
```

# Layered Raspberries, Bing Cherries, and Oranges

*This is an easy-to-make but elegant dessert. Fresh raspberries, sweet dark cherries, and sliced navel oranges are marinated in cherry-flavored fruit juice and then layered in chilled stemmed glasses. To remove the pits from the cherries easily, use a cherry pitter. This small, inexpensive tool can be purchased at cookware stores. If not available, cut cherries in half and remove pits.*

YIELD: 5 c (1¼ qt) fruit                                SERVINGS: 8
SERVING SIZE: ⅝ c fruit

|  | WEIGHT | MEASURE |
|---|---|---|
| Navel oranges | 18 oz as purchased | 2 large |
| Bing cherries | 12 oz as purchased | 2½ c (1¼ pt) |
| Fresh ripe raspberries | 6 oz as purchased | 1¼ c |
| Thawed white grape juice concentrate, undiluted |  | ¼ c + 2 tbsp |
| Cherry extract |  | 1½ tsp |

Peel oranges with a small sharp knife. Cut away any remaining bits of white pith. Cut in half lengthwise. Cut across into thin half-rounds. Place in a small storage container.

Wash cherries and remove stems and pits. Place in a small storage container.

Wash raspberries and place in a small storage container.

Combine juice concentrate and cherry extract in a small bowl. Mix until blended. Pour ⅓ juice mixture over each fruit. Cover and refrigerate for at least 2 hours, basting occasionally with marinade.

Layer oranges, cherries, and raspberries in 8 chilled stemmed glasses, topping with an orange slice. Ladle any remaining marinade over fruit and serve.

---

### NUTRITIONAL FACTS

| | | |
|---|---|---|
| Calories: 99 (5% from fat) | Carbohydrate: 22.9 g and | Iron: .4 mg |
| Fat: .6 g (.1 g sat, .1 g | 86% | Sodium: 1.6 mg |
| mono, .2 g poly) | Alcohol: .6 g and 4% | Calcium: 38.3 mg |
| Protein: 1.5 g and 5% | Fiber: 4 g | Diabetic Exchanges: 1½ |
| | Cholesterol: 0 mg | Fruits |

---

# Minted Melon Balls Marinated in Fruit Juice Syrup

*According to Greek mythology, Persephone, wife of Pluto, was so jealous of a nymph named Mentha that the goddess turned her into the lowly mint plant. In this recipe, the fragrant herb contributes a refreshing zip to a medley of chilled melon balls that have been gently tossed in a citrus juice, honey, and currant jelly glaze.*

YIELD: 3 c (1½ pt) melon balls          SERVINGS: 6
SERVING SIZE: ½ c melon balls

| | WEIGHT | MEASURE |
|---|---|---|
| Currant jelly | | 1½ tbsp |
| Honey | | 1 tbsp |
| Fresh orange juice | | ¼ c |
| Fresh lemon juice | | 1½ tbsp |
| Fresh lime juice | | 1 tbsp |
| Minced mint leaves | | 1 tbsp |
| Assorted ½-inch melon balls such as can-<br>taloupe, honeydew, and seedless water-<br>melon | 1 lb | 3 c (1½ pt) |

Combine currant jelly and honey in a small saucepan. Heat to a boil, stir-ring. Remove from heat. Set aside to cool a few minutes. When cool, stir in orange, lemon, and lime juices and mint leaves. Pour syrup over melon balls. Cover and refrigerate until chilled. Spoon into 6 chilled stemmed glasses or dessert dishes. Garnish with mint sprigs, if desired, and serve.

---

### NUTRITIONAL FACTS

Calories: 54 (5% from fat)
Fat: .4 g (0 g sat, .1 g
   mono, .1 g poly)
Protein: .6 g and 4%

Carbohydrate: 13.2 g and
   91%
Fiber: .4 g
Cholesterol: 0 mg
Iron: .2 mg

Sodium: 4.3 mg
Calcium: 8 mg
Diabetic Exchanges:
   ½ Other Carbohydrate;
   ½ Fruit

# Navel Oranges and Kiwis Sprinkled with Berries in Rose-Scented Syrup

*The pleasing, tangy flavor of naval oranges and their lack of seeds are reasons enough to eat this citrus fruit. But there are more. Navel oranges are rich in vitamin C, folic acid, and fiber, too.* Nutrition Action Healthletter *lists oranges as number one of the ten super foods you should eat. Naval oranges can be identified by the navel-like appearance of their blossom ends. When selecting oranges of all types, choose firm heavy ones. The heavier they are for their size, the juicier they will be. Refrigerated, oranges store well for several weeks.*

*In this recipe, peeled and sliced navel oranges and kiwis are layered and then drizzled with rose-perfumed honey. To finish the dish, strawberries and blueberries are sprinkled over. The secret to this colorful fruit medley's fragrance is rose water, a distillation of rose petals. It is available in ethnic and specialty markets. Don't reserve rose water for just fresh fruit desserts, though. Enhance salad dressings, stews, soups, rice pilafs, pastries, and dinner coffees with a splash, too.*

YIELD: 6 c (1½ qt) fruit

SERVINGS: 12

SERVING SIZE: ½ c fruit

|  | WEIGHT | MEASURE |
|---|---|---|
| Honey |  | 2 tbsp |
| Rose water |  | 1 tsp |
| Navel oranges | 2 lb as purchased | 4 large |
| Kiwis | 12 oz as purchased | 4 medium |
| Fresh ripe strawberries, hulled | 5 oz as purchased | 1 c |
| Fresh ripe blueberries | 5 oz as purchased | 1 c |

Combine honey and rose water in a small bowl. Mix until blended.

Remove peel from oranges with a small sharp knife. Cut away any remaining bits of white pith. Cut oranges in half lengthwise. Cut across into very thin half-rounds. If there are any seeds, remove them. Arrange in a 1½-quart glass serving bowl or 12 stemmed glasses.

Cut off both ends of kiwis. Remove skin with a vegetable peeler or small sharp knife. Cut in half lengthwise, then into thin half-rounds. Arrange over oranges.

Drizzle honey mixture over fruit. Tilt bowl or glasses to baste fruit with accumulated juice. Refrigerate until chilled.

Cut strawberries lengthwise into thin slices, then into narrow strips. Wash blueberries. Sprinkle strawberries and blueberries over oranges and kiwis and serve.

---

### NUTRITIONAL FACTS

Calories: 74 (3% from fat)
Fat: .3 g (0 g sat, 0 g
   mono, .1 g poly)
Protein: 1.2 g and 6%

Carbohydrate: 18.4 g and
   90%
Alcohol: .1 and 1%
Fiber: 5.1 g
Cholesterol: 0 mg

Iron: .3 mg
Sodium: 3.2 mg
Calcium: 40.2 mg
Diabetic Exchanges: 1
   Fruit

---

# Orange Sections in Raspberry Syrup Splashed with Chambord

*To the delight of many, the USDA Dietary Guidelines for Americans state that alcohol not only can enhance meals but also might have health benefits if consumed in moderation. While the benefits of moderate alcohol consumption may be news to many, the culinary world discovered its merits long ago. In this recipe, a splash of Chambord, the cognac-based raspberry liqueur, elevates the "common" orange to new heights.*

YIELD: 2½ c (1¼ pt) orange sections      SERVINGS: 5
SERVING SIZE: ½ c orange sections

|  | WEIGHT | MEASURE |
|---|---|---|
| 100%-fruit raspberry spread | 3 oz | ¼ c |
| Chambord or other raspberry liqueur |  | 2 tbsp |
| Navel or Valencia orange sections (6 medium) | 1 lb sections | 2½ c (1¼ pt) |

Combine raspberry spread and Chambord in a small bowl. Mix until blended.

Pour syrup over orange sections. Cover. Refrigerate until oranges are permeated with raspberry flavor, or about 3 hours. Spoon into 5 chilled dessert dishes or stemmed glasses and serve.

---

### NUTRITIONAL FACTS

| | | |
|---|---|---|
| Calories: 120 (2% from fat) | Carbohydrate: 28 g and 87% | Sodium: 2.2 mg |
| Fat: .2 g (0 g sat, 0 g mono, .1 g poly) | Alcohol: 1.1 g and 6% | Calcium: 96.6 mg |
| Protein: 1.7 g and 5% | Fiber: 4.7 g | Diabetic Exchanges: ½ Other Carbohydrate; 1½ Fruits |
| | Cholesterol: 0 mg | |
| | Iron: .9 mg | |

---

# Papaya Banana Sauce Sweetened with Fruit Juice

*This recipe began as frozen yogurt. In the process of creating the dessert, I took a taste of this creamy and smooth, sweet, yet slightly tart and exotic-flavored papaya banana purée and the rest is history. Papayas are harvested when only one-fourth ripe, so set them at room temperature to ripen completely. The papayas are ripe and ready to use when they yield slightly to palm pressure. Refrigerate ripe fruit and use as soon as possible.*

YIELD: 3 c (1½ pt) sauce            SERVINGS: 6
SERVING SIZE: ½ c sauce

| | WEIGHT | MEASURE |
|---|---|---|
| Ripe peeled papaya cubes | 18 oz | 3½ c (1¾ pt) |
| Very ripe peeled banana slices | 6 oz | 1 c |
| Thawed white grape juice concentrate, undiluted | | ¼ c + 2 tbsp |

Combine all ingredients in a food processor or blender. Blend until smooth. Spoon into 6 dessert dishes and serve at room temperature or chilled.

<table>
<tr><td colspan="3" align="center">NUTRITIONAL FACTS</td></tr>
<tr>
<td>Calories: 91 (3% from fat)<br>Fat: .3 g (.1 g sat, .1 g<br>   mono, .1 g poly)<br>Protein: .9 g and 4%</td>
<td>Carbohydrate: 23 g and<br>   93%<br>Fiber: 2.3 g<br>Cholesterol: 0 mg<br>Iron: .2 mg</td>
<td>Sodium: 4.1 mg<br>Calcium: 24.5 mg<br>Diabetic Exchanges: 1½<br>   Fruits</td>
</tr>
</table>

# Pineapple Wedges Decorated with Melon Balls

*Unlike bananas and pears, once pineapples are picked they may grow softer and juicier but won't get sweeter. They lack a reserve of starch for conversion to sugar. To select a ripe pineapple, choose one that is large, plump, and fresh looking with crisp, uniformly green leaves and a sweet fragrance. Don't rely on the color of the fruit's shell to indicate ripeness. It may vary from green to golden. Contrary to popular belief, pulling a leaf from the fruit's crown and thumping won't tell you if it's ripe.*

YIELD: 1 pineapple                   SERVINGS: 8
SERVING SIZE: one-eighth pineapple

|  | WEIGHT | MEASURE |
| --- | --- | --- |
| Ripe pineapple, chilled | 5 lb as purchased | 1 large |
| Ripe cantaloupe, chilled | 12 oz as purchased | one-fourth 3-lb melon |
| Ripe honeydew, chilled | 12 oz as purchased | one-eighth 6-lb melon |

Cut pineapple lengthwise into 8 wedges with a heavy knife, cutting evenly through leaves and core. Cut fruit from shell with a sharp curved knife, then cut away core. Cut fruit crosswise into equally spaced bite-size chunks (about 7). Slide fruit chunks ½ inch in alternating directions so chunks extend alternately to one side then other.

Cut melons in half and remove seeds. Cut into balls by pressing large end of a melon baller deep into flesh, twisting and removing. Place cantaloupe and honeydew balls alternately on top of pineapple chunks. Serve on 8 chilled plates.

---

### NUTRITIONAL FACTS

Calories: 105 (5% from fat)

Fat: .6 g (.1 g sat, .1 g mono, .2 g poly)

Protein: 1.2 g and 4%

Carbohydrate: 26.2 g and 91%

Fiber: 2 g

Cholesterol: 0 mg

Iron: .7 mg

Sodium: 16.4 mg

Calcium: 18.8 mg

Diabetic Exchanges: 2 Fruits

---

# Sliced Strawberries Macerated in Port

*Port is a sweet fortified wine. There are many different types so select one that best fits your budget and your taste buds. Usually rich and fruity in flavor, ruby ports are the very youngest ports. Tawny ports are much smoother than ruby ports, and have just a touch of sweetness. Vintage ports are by far the best ports but also the most expensive. They are made from the grapes of a single vintage and bottled within two years.*

YIELD: 2½ c (1¼ pt) strawberries　　　　　　　　SERVINGS: 5
SERVING SIZE: ½ c strawberries

| | WEIGHT | MEASURE |
|---|---|---|
| Hulled and sliced fresh ripe strawberries | 15 oz | 2½ c (1¼ pt) |
| Port or other sweet wine | | 3 tbsp |
| Thawed white grape juice concentrate, undiluted | | 1 tbsp |

Place berries in a small storage container.

Combine port and juice concentrate in a small bowl. Mix until blended. Pour over berries. Toss gently to coat. Refrigerate to marinate 12 hours.

Spoon berries into 5 chilled dessert dishes. Garnish with mint sprigs, if desired, and serve.

---

### NUTRITIONAL FACTS

| | | |
|---|---|---|
| Calories: 39 (6% from fat) | Carbohydrate: 7 g and 66% | Iron: .3 mg |
| Fat: .3 g (0 g sat, 0 g mono, .2 g poly) | Alcohol: 1.4 g and 22% | Sodium: 1.7 mg |
| Protein: .5 g and 5% | Fiber: 1.8 g | Calcium: 12 mg |
| | Cholesterol: 0 mg | Diabetic Exchanges: ½ Fruit |

# Summer Fruit Layered with Vanilla Amaretto Custard Sauce

*Three different methods are described in this recipe to present this colorful array of fresh sliced fruit and creamy smooth vanilla sauce. But the list is endless, so try one of these or create your own.*

YIELD: 5 c (1¼ qt) fruit + 2 c (1 pt) sauce     SERVINGS: 8
SERVING SIZE: ⅝ c fruit + ¼ c sauce

| | WEIGHT | MEASURE |
|---|---|---|
| Peeled and thinly sliced peaches, chilled | 6 oz | 1 c |
| Hulled and sliced fresh ripe strawberries, chilled | 6 oz | 1 c |
| Peeled and sliced kiwis (about 3 large), chilled | 6 oz | 1 c |
| Seedless green grape halves, chilled | 6 oz | 1 c |
| Fresh ripe blackberries, chilled | 6 oz | 1 c |
| Creamy Vanilla Custard Sauce Spiked with Amaretto (page 215), chilled | | 1 recipe |

To peel peaches, blanch them in boiling water for 20 to 60 seconds and then place in ice water or under cold running water until completely cooled. The skins should slip off easily.

Layer fruit with sauce in 8 chilled stemmed glasses ending with fruit on top. Or, swirl sauce on 8 chilled dessert plates and then decorate with fruit. Or, arrange fruit attractively in 8 chilled dessert dishes and spoon sauce over. Garnish with mint sprigs, if desired, and serve immediately.

---

### NUTRITIONAL FACTS

Calories: 173 (12% from fat)

Fat: 2.3 g (.9 g sat, .7 g mono, .4 g poly)

Protein: 5.2 g and 12%

Carbohydrate: 34.1 g and 76%

Alcohol: .3 g and 1%

Fiber: 2.9 g

Cholesterol: 55.6 mg

Iron: .7 mg

Sodium: 63.4 mg

Calcium: 100.1 mg

Diabetic Exchanges: 1 Other Carbohydrate; 1 Fruit; ½ Low-Fat Milk

# Watermelon and Raspberries in Light Raspberry Glaze

*Watermelon is loved by both kids and adults. For a refreshing finish to a meal, gently toss seedless bright red watermelon balls with ruby-red raspberries and finish with a drizzle of white grape juice concentrate and a splash of raspberry vinegar. Like a squeeze of lemon juice on broccoli, the raspberry vinegar brightens the natural flavor of both the watermelon and raspberries in this recipe.*

YIELD: 4 c (1 qt) fruit                                    SERVINGS: 8
SERVING SIZE: ½ c fruit

|  | WEIGHT | MEASURE |
|---|---|---|
| Thawed white grape juice concentrate, undiluted |  | ¼ c |
| Raspberry vinegar |  | 1 tbsp |
| ½-inch balls or cubes seedless watermelon | 1 lb | 3 c (1½ pt) |
| Fresh ripe raspberries | 4 oz | 1 c |

Combine juice concentrate and vinegar in a small bowl. Mix to blend.

Combine melon balls and raspberries in a medium bowl. Pour juice mixture over fruit. Mix gently until fruit is well coated with sauce. Spoon into 8 dessert dishes or stemmed glasses. Garnish with mint sprigs, if desired, and serve.

---

### NUTRITIONAL FACTS

Calories: 30 (9% from fat)
Fat: .3 g (0 g sat, .1 g mono, .1 g poly)
Protein: .5 g and 6%

Carbohydrate: 7 g and 85%
Fiber: 1.3 g
Cholesterol: 0 mg
Iron: .2 mg

Sodium: 1.3 mg
Calcium: 8 mg
Diabetic Exchanges: ½ Fruit

# Fruit Crisps, Crumbles, Tortes, Sauces, and Other Cooked Fruit Desserts and Gelatins

Apple Crisp with Brown Sugar Oat Topping

Baked Applesauce Sprinkled with Toasted Fennel Seeds

Baked Banana Peach Crumble with Gingersnap Topping

Baked Pear Halves Stuffed with Dates in Aromatic Orange Syrup

Date and Almond-Stuffed Baked Apples

Fresh Pear Torte Laced with Dried Cranberries

Granny Smith and Red Plum Applesauce

Juicy Pineapple Cubes in Spicy Sweet Marinade

Meringue-Topped Blueberry Stuffed Poached Peach Halves

Peach Blackberry Crumble with Whole Wheat Topping

Peanut Butter and Jelly Apple Rings Topped with Meringue

Purple Plum Blueberry Oat Crunch

Rhubarb Compote Laced with Dried Cranberries

Rum-Flavored Sour Cream Gelatin Dotted with Peaches

Sweet Tofu and Yogurt Gelatin with Strawberry Bits

# Apple Crisp with Brown Sugar Oat Topping

*There are more than just red and green apples to choose from today. But of the thousands of varieties, only about twenty are readily available. Green, tart, and crisp Granny Smith apples are great for eating raw but taste equally good stuffed, baked whole, or sliced and cooked in desserts like this crisp. It's no wonder these all-purpose apples rank third in popularity nationwide.*

YIELD: 8-inch square crisp                                      SERVINGS: 9
SERVING SIZE: 2⅔-inch square

|  | WEIGHT | MEASURE |
|---|---|---|
| Firmly packed light brown sugar, divided | 3 oz | 6 tbsp |
| Honey, divided |  | 2 tbsp |
| Firmly packed raisins | 2 oz | ⅓ c |
| Cornstarch | 1 oz | 3½ tbsp |
| Ground cinnamon |  | 1 tsp |
| Finely grated orange zest |  | ½ tsp |
| Ground nutmeg |  | ¼ tsp |
| Peeled, cored, and thinly sliced Granny Smith or other tart apples | 1¼ lb | 4½ c (1⅛ qt) |
| Long-cooking ("old-fashioned") rolled oats | 3 oz | 1 c |
| Whole wheat flour | 2 oz | ½ c |
| Stick margarine, chilled | 1 oz | 2 tbsp |

Preheat oven to 350 degrees F.

Combine 3 tablespoons (1½ ounces) brown sugar, 1 tablespoon honey, raisins, cornstarch, cinnamon, orange zest, and nutmeg in a medium bowl. Mix until well blended. Add apples. Toss gently until well coated. Spoon into an 8-inch square baking pan.

Combine oats, flour, margarine, and remaining 3 tablespoons brown sugar and 1 tablespoon honey in a small bowl. Work mixture with a pastry blender or your fingertips until crumbly.

Sprinkle crumbs over apple mixture. Bake until apples are tender, or about 1 hour. If top is becoming too brown after 30 minutes, cover loosely with foil and continue baking. Cut into 9 squares. Top with a scoop of vanilla reduced-fat ice cream, if desired, and serve warm.

# Baked Applesauce Sprinkled with Toasted Fennel Seeds

*Apples may be better than vitamin C in preventing cancer, according to scientists from Cornell University and Seoul National University. In a report published in the* Lancet *medical journal, the researchers credit quercetin, a natural phytochemical found in apples, for the anticancer activity. In this sugar-free recipe, sliced apples are baked with apple juice concentrate, then puréed and seasoned with cinnamon, ginger, nutmeg, and a sprinkle of toasted fennel seeds.*

YIELD: 2½ c (1¼ pt) applesauce                    SERVINGS: 5
SERVING SIZE: ½ c applesauce

| | WEIGHT | MEASURE |
|---|---|---|
| Apple juice | | ½ c |
| Lemon juice | | 1 tbsp |
| Cooking apples, cored | 2 lb | 6 medium |
| Thawed apple juice concentrate, undiluted | | ¼ c + 2 tbsp |
| Ground cinnamon | | 1 tsp |
| Ground ginger | | ¼ tsp |
| Ground nutmeg | | ¼ tsp |
| Fennel seeds, toasted and crushed | | 2 tsp |

Preheat oven to 375 degrees F.

Combine apple and lemon juices in a 13-by-9-by-2-inch baking pan. Slice apples into juices, to prevent browning. Cover and bake, stirring occasionally, until apples are tender but not mushy, or about 30 minutes.

Spoon apples into a food processor or blender. Add apple juice concentrate, cinnamon, ginger, and nutmeg. Blend until smooth. Strain through a fine mesh strainer to remove peels. Spoon into 5 dessert dishes. Sprinkle with toasted fennel seeds and serve warm, at room temperature, or chilled. To toast seeds, cook in a dry nonstick skillet over medium heat, stirring constantly until fragrant, or 2 to 3 minutes.

### NUTRITIONAL FACTS

| | | |
|---|---|---|
| Calories: 133 (5% from fat) | Protein: .5 g and 1% | Iron: .7 mg |
| Fat: .8 g (.1 g sat, .1 g mono, .2 g poly) | Carbohydrate: 33.9 g and 93% | Sodium: 5.9 mg |
| | Fiber: 3.6 g | Calcium: 27 mg |
| | Cholesterol: 0 mg | Diabetic Exchanges: 2 Fruits |

# Baked Banana Peach Crumble with Gingersnap Topping

*Technically, this is a Brown Betty (fruit layered and topped with sweet buttered crumbs) but the term "crumble" seemed more appropriate for this dessert. A "crumble" is defined as a fruit mixture topped with an all-flour streusel. Warm out of the oven, topped with a scoop of vanilla fat-free frozen yogurt just beginning to melt, this crumble is ready to "crumble."*

YIELD: 8-inch square crumble
SERVING SIZE: 2⅔-inch square

SERVINGS: 9

| | WEIGHT | MEASURE |
|---|---|---|
| Butter-flavored vegetable oil cooking spray | — | — |
| ⅛-inch-thick slices peeled ripe peaches | 18 oz | 3 c (1½ pt) |
| Stick margarine | 1½ oz | 3 tbsp |
| Gingersnap crumbs | 10½ oz | 2½ c (1¼ pt) |
| Cornstarch | | 1⅓ tbsp |
| Thawed white grape juice concentrate, undiluted | | ¼ c |
| Thawed orange juice concentrate, undiluted | | 2 tbsp |
| Light rum (or ¾ tsp rum extract) | | 1 tbsp |
| ¼-inch-thick slices peeled ripe bananas | 18 oz | scant 3½ c (about 4 large bananas) |

Preheat oven to 350 degrees F. Coat an 8-inch square baking pan with cooking spray.

To peel peaches, blanch them in boiling water for 20 to 60 seconds, then place in ice water or under cold running water until completely cooled. The skins should slip off easily.

Melt margarine in a medium saucepan over low heat. Remove from heat. Add gingersnap crumbs. Stir to mix.

Combine cornstarch, grape and orange juice concentrates, and rum in a small bowl. Mix until smooth.

Layer half bananas, half peaches, and half gingersnap crumbs in prepared baking pan. Top with remaining bananas and peaches. Pour juice concentrate mixture over. Sprinkle remaining gingersnap crumbs over.

Bake until fruit is tender, or about 20 minutes. Cut into 9 squares. Top with a scoop of vanilla fat-free frozen yogurt, if desired, and serve warm.

---

### NUTRITIONAL FACTS

Calories: 272 (24% from fat)

Fat: 7.4 g (1.7 g sat, 3.6 g mono, 1.7 g poly)

Protein: 3 g and 4%

Carbohydrate: 50.5 g and 72%

Alcohol: .2 g and 0%

Fiber: 3.2 g

Cholesterol: 0 mg

Iron: 2.4 mg

Sodium: 217.8 mg

Calcium: 34.5 mg

Diabetic Exchanges: ½ Starch; 1½ Other Carbohydrates; 1½ Fruits; 1½ Fats

# Baked Pear Halves Stuffed with Dates in Aromatic Orange Syrup

*There are two primary types of pears: the European pear with its soft and succulent flesh, yellow or red skin, and pear shape, and the Asian pear with its crunchy flesh, green-yellow or russet skin, and round shape. Select the European variety for this recipe. Firm yet ripe, Anjou, Bartlett, Bosc, or Comice pears make excellent choices.*

YIELD: 8 stuffed pear halves          SERVING SIZE: ½ stuffed pear

| | WEIGHT | MEASURE |
|---|---|---|
| Fresh ripe pears | 22 oz | 4 medium |
| Coarsely chopped seedless dates | 4 oz | ¾ c |
| Chopped walnuts | 1 oz | ¼ c |
| Finely grated orange zest | | 1 tsp |
| Fresh orange juice | | 1 c |
| Honey | 4½ oz | ¼ c + 2 tbsp |
| Ground cinnamon | | ⅛ tsp |
| Ground nutmeg | | ⅛ tsp |
| Ground cloves | | ⅛ tsp |

Preheat oven to 350 degrees F.

Peel pears and cut in half lengthwise. Core and scoop out a bit extra to make a cavity. Cut a small slice off each pear's rounded side so it sits flat. Place in a baking pan. Chop pear cuttings into small pieces.

Combine chopped pears, dates, walnuts, and orange zest in a small bowl. Mix until blended. Spoon mixture into pears' cavities.

Combine orange juice, honey, cinnamon, nutmeg, and cloves in a small bowl. Mix until blended. Pour over pears.

Cover and bake until pears are tender, or about 25 minutes, basting occasionally with orange juice syrup. Spoon into 8 dessert dishes and serve warm, at room temperature, or chilled.

| NUTRITIONAL FACTS | | |
|---|---|---|
| Calories: 173 (13% from fat) | Carbohydrate: 40 g and 84% | Sodium: 1.8 mg |
| Fat: 2.7 g (.3 g sat, .6 g mono, 1.5 g poly) | Fiber: 4 g | Calcium: 22.5 mg |
| Protein: 1.4 g and 3% | Cholesterol: 0 mg | Diabetic Exchanges: 1 |
| | Iron: .6 mg | Other Carbohydrate; 1½ Fruits; ½ Fat |

# Date and Almond-Stuffed Baked Apples

*For best results, prepare this recipe with uniform-sized apples that stay firm and flavorful when baked. Good choices include Baldwin, Cortland, Northern Spy, Rome Beauty, Winesap, and York Imperial apples. Always store apples in the coldest part of the refrigerator. They deteriorate faster at room temperature.*

YIELD: 8 stuffed apples          SERVING SIZE: 1 stuffed apple

| | WEIGHT | MEASURE |
|---|---|---|
| Slivered almonds, chopped and toasted without fat | 1 oz | ¼ c |
| Baking apples, cored | 3 lb as purchased | 8 medium |
| Chopped seedless dates | 2 oz | ¼ c + 2 tbsp |
| Natural wheat and barley cereal (such as Grape Nuts) | 2 oz | ½ c |
| Lemon juice | | 2 tsp |
| Ground cinnamon | | ½ tsp |
| Ground nutmeg | | ¼ tsp |
| Maple syrup, divided | | ½ c |
| Apple juice | | ¾ c |

Preheat oven to 350 degrees F. To toast almonds, cook in a dry nonstick skillet over medium heat, stirring constantly until they just begin to become fragrant, or about 4 minutes.

Slice a little off bottoms of apples as needed so they sit flat. Place in a 13-by-9-by-2-inch baking pan.

Combine almonds, dates, cereal, lemon juice, cinnamon, nutmeg, and ¼ cup maple syrup in a small bowl. Mix until well blended. Spoon filling into cavities of apples, dividing evenly. Pack lightly. Pour remaining ¼ cup maple syrup and apple juice around apples.

Cover and bake for 30 minutes. Uncover and continue baking, basting with juice-syrup mixture until tender when pierced with a pointed knife, or about 25 minutes. Spoon into 8 dessert dishes. Ladle syrup over and serve warm, at room temperature, or chilled.

### NUTRITIONAL FACTS

| | | |
|---|---|---|
| Calories: 212 (10% from fat) | Carbohydrate: 49.2 g and 86% | Sodium: 52.1 mg |
| Fat: 2.5 g (.3 g sat, 1.2 g mono, .5 g poly) | Fiber: 5.5 g | Calcium: 41 mg |
| Protein: 2.1 g and 4% | Cholesterol: 0 mg | Diabetic Exchanges: ½ Starch; ½ Other Carbohydrate; 2 Fruits; ½ Fat |
| | Iron: 2.7 mg | |

# Fresh Pear Torte Laced with Dried Cranberries

*Of the more than five thousand varieties of pears grown throughout the world, this dessert calls for the familiar, bell-shaped, yellow-green to dark red-skinned, sweet, juicy, smooth fleshed Bartlett pear. Unlike most fruits, the pear's texture and flavor improve after it's picked. For this recipe, select pears that are fragrant and free of blemishes and soft spots. If purchased firm, store them in a loosely closed paper bag at room temperature until they are ripe or give to gentle pressure. Ripe unwashed pears can be refrigerated for up to three days.*

YIELD: 9-inch torte                                    SERVINGS: 16
SERVING SIZE: 1 wedge (one-sixteenth 9-inch torte)

| | WEIGHT | MEASURE |
| --- | --- | --- |
| Butter-flavored vegetable oil cooking spray | — | — |
| Large eggs | 4 oz | 2 |
| Firmly packed light brown sugar, divided | 7 oz | ¾ c + 2 tbsp |
| Whole wheat pastry flour or whole wheat flour | 6 oz | 1 ⅓ c |
| Baking powder | | 2 tsp |
| Finely grated lemon zest | | ¾ tsp |
| Finely grated orange zest | | ¾ tsp |
| Fat-free milk | | ⅔ c |
| Peeled, cored, and thinly sliced ripe Bartlett pears | 2¼ lb as purchased | 5 c (1¼ qt) |
| Sweetened dried cranberries or cherries | 3 oz | scant ⅔ c |

Preheat oven to 350 degrees F. Coat a 9-inch springform pan with cooking spray.

Place eggs in a medium bowl. Whisk until blended. Add 6 ounces (¾ cup) brown sugar. Whisk until well blended. Add flour, baking powder, and lemon and orange zests. Mix until blended. Slowly add milk, mixing until just blended. Let stand 15 minutes.

Pour batter into prepared springform pan. Combine pears and cranberries in a bowl. Gently toss until mixed. Arrange pear-cranberry mixture attractively over batter, pressing down so all fruit fits in pan. Sprinkle with remaining 1 ounce (2 tablespoons) brown sugar.

Bake until pears are tender and torte is firm to the touch, or about 1 hour and 20 to 30 minutes. If top is becoming too brown, cover loosely with foil.

Cool torte in pan on a rack for 5 minutes. Run a knife around edge of pan and release sides. Place on a plate. Rearrange any pear slices that are out of place. Sift powdered sugar over, if desired, and serve warm.

| NUTRITIONAL FACTS | | |
|---|---|---|
| Calories: 141 (7% from fat) | Carbohydrate: 31.9 g and 86% | Sodium: 80 mg |
| Fat: 1.1 g (.3 g sat, .3 g mono, .2 g poly) | Fiber: 2.8 g | Calcium: 70.2 mg |
| | Cholesterol: 26.8 mg | Diabetic Exchanges: ½ |
| Protein: 2.8 g and 8% | Iron: 1 mg | Starch; ½ Other Carbo-hydrate; 1 Fruit |

# Granny Smith and Red Plum Applesauce

*Granny Smith apples and red plums are the secret to the irresistibly sweet yet slightly tart flavor of this smooth and rosy-hued applesauce. Replace the Granny Smith apples and red plums with other varieties of apples and plums when those are not available. Simply increase or decrease the amount of apple juice concentrate called for in the recipe as needed to adjust for the tartness of the apples and plums selected.*

YIELD: 5 c (1 ¼ qt) sauce  SERVINGS: 10
SERVING SIZE: ½ c sauce

|  | WEIGHT | MEASURE |
|---|---|---|
| Granny Smith or other tart apples | 2 lb as purchased | 6 medium |
| Red plums | 1 lb as purchased | 12 to 15 |
| Thawed apple juice concentrate, undiluted | | 1 c |
| Water | | ½ c |
| Whole cloves | | 2 |
| Cinnamon stick | | ½-inch piece |
| Lemon juice | | 2 tsp |
| Ground nutmeg | | pinch |

Core apples and cut into chunks. Pit plums and cut into chunks. Place in a large saucepan. Add apple juice concentrate, water, cloves, and cinnamon stick. (Place cloves and cinnamon stick in a cheesecloth bag for easy removal if desired.) Heat to boiling, then reduce heat to low. Simmer, covered, stirring occasionally, until plums and apples are tender, or about 20 minutes.

Remove cloves and cinnamon from apple mixture. Process fruit in a blender or food processor until puréed. Press through a fine mesh strainer to remove fruit skins.

Stir in lemon juice and nutmeg. Taste. For a sweeter sauce, flavor with additional apple juice concentrate. (It will not be included in the nutritional facts.) Spoon into 10 dessert dishes and serve warm, at room temperature, or chilled, or as a topping for breakfast items such as whole grain pancakes and waffles.

---

### NUTRITIONAL FACTS

| | | |
|---|---|---|
| Calories: 126 (5% from fat) | Carbohydrate: 31.4 g and 93% | Sodium: 7.2 mg |
| Fat: .7 g (.1 g sat, .2 g mono, .2 g poly) | Fiber: 2.8 g | Calcium: 15.5 mg |
| Protein: .7 g and 2% | Cholesterol: 0 mg | Diabetic Exchanges: 2 Fruits |
| | Iron: .5 mg | |

---

# Juicy Pineapple Cubes in Spicy Sweet Marinade

*These naturally sweet and juicy pineapple cubes might be described as aromatic edible jewels—with a little bite. Steeping the cubes in a fruit juice and vinegar marinade and seasoning them with cinnamon, clove, cardamom, and a pinch of red pepper effects the transformation. This sauce can be served both as a topping for reduced-fat ice creams and cakes or as an accompaniment with poultry and fish selections.*

YIELD: 3 c (1½ pt) pineapple cubes          SERVINGS: 6
SERVING SIZE: ½ c pineapple cubes

| | WEIGHT | MEASURE |
|---|---|---|
| Ripe pineapple | 3½ lb | 1 medium |
| Pineapple juice from fresh pineapple or water | | 1 c |
| Apple cider vinegar | | ½ c |
| Thawed pineapple juice concentrate, undiluted | | ½ c |
| Thawed white grape juice concentrate, undiluted | | ¼ c |
| Cinnamon stick | | 3-inch piece |
| Whole cloves | | 1 tsp |
| Lightly crushed whole cardamom pods | | 1 tsp |
| Whole allspice | | ¼ tsp |
| Crushed red pepper flakes | | pinch |

Peel, core, and cut pineapple into ½-inch cubes, reserving as much juice as possible. Or use 1½ pounds (3 cups) fresh or frozen and thawed unsweetened pineapple cubes and 1 cup pineapple juice. Place cubes in a storage container. Set aside.

Combine pineapple juice, vinegar, juice concentrates, cinnamon stick, cloves, cardamom, allspice, and red pepper flakes in a small saucepan. Heat to boiling, then reduce heat to low. Cover and simmer for 15 minutes.

Ladle spicy fruit juice over pineapple cubes. Cool. Cover tightly and refrigerate for at least 24 hours. Spoon into 6 dessert dishes and serve, or offer as a topping for angel food cake or vanilla reduced-fat ice cream.

---

### NUTRITIONAL FACTS

Calories: 135 (4% from fat)

Fat: .6 g (.1 g sat, .1 g mono, .2 g poly)

Protein: .9 g and 3%

Carbohydrate: 33.7 g and 93%

Fiber: 1.6 g

Cholesterol: 0 mg

Iron: .9 mg

Sodium: 8.1 mg

Calcium: 25.6 mg

Diabetic Exchanges: 2½ Fruits

---

# Meringue-Topped Blueberry Stuffed Poached Peach Halves

*Fat- and cholesterol-free egg white meringue transforms these peach halves stuffed with ripe and juicy blueberries into an elegant dessert. To peel a peach or two for eating, use a vegetable peeler or small sharp knife. To save time when peeling more than a couple of peaches, blanch the peaches in boiling water for 20 to 60 seconds and then place them in ice water or under cold running water until completely cooled. The skins should slip off easily.*

YIELD: 8 peach halves          SERVING SIZE: ½ peach

|  | WEIGHT | MEASURE |
| --- | --- | --- |
| Fresh ripe peaches, peeled, halved, and pitted | 24 oz as purchased | 4 medium |
| Fresh or frozen unsweetened blueberries | 3 oz | ⅔ c |
| Granulated sugar, divided | 4 oz | ½ c |
| Finely grated orange zest |  | 1 tsp |
| Thawed orange juice concentrate, undiluted |  | ½ c |
| Water |  | ½ c |
| Large egg whites, at room temperature | 2½ oz | 2 |
| Cream of tartar |  | ⅛ tsp |
| Vanilla extract |  | ½ tsp |

Preheat oven to 350 degrees F.

Scoop out center of each peach half to form a cavity. Cut a small slice off each peach's rounded side so it sits flat. Chop center and end pieces into small bits. Place peach halves, cut side up, in a shallow baking pan or individual baking ramekins. Combine chopped peaches, blueberries, 2 ounces (¼ cup) sugar, and orange zest in a small bowl. Mix together. Spoon mixture into peach cavities.

Combine orange juice concentrate and water in a small bowl. Mix until blended. Pour around peach halves. Cover and bake until peaches are tender, or about 25 minutes. Remove from oven and set aside. Increase oven temperature to 400 degrees F.

Combine egg whites and cream of tartar in a medium mixing bowl. Beat with an electric mixer until whites hold soft peaks. Gradually add remaining 2 ounces (¼ cup) sugar, continuing to beat until stiff peaks form. Beat in vanilla until incorporated.

Spoon meringue over top of each peach half, dividing evenly. Bake, uncovered, until meringue is golden brown, or 3 to 5 minutes. Spoon into 8 dessert dishes and serve warm, at room temperature, or chilled.

---

### NUTRITIONAL FACTS

| | | |
|---|---|---|
| Calories: 123 (1% from fat) | Carbohydrate: 30 g and 93% | Sodium: 15.5 mg |
| Fat: .1 g (0 g sat, 0 g mono, .1 g poly) | Fiber: 1.8 g | Calcium: 11 mg |
| Protein: 1.8 g and 6% | Cholesterol: 0 mg | Diabetic Exchanges: 1 |
| | Iron: .2 mg | Other Carbohydrate; 1 Fruit |

---

# Peach Blackberry Crumble with Whole Wheat Topping

*Pandowdies, cobblers, crumbles, and crunches all begin with sweetened fruit. It's their topping that determines their name. Properly speaking, when fruit is baked topped with spoonfuls of biscuit batter, it's a cobbler, and a pandowdy when the topping is rolled-out biscuit dough. A crumble is topped with an all-flour streusel and a crunch with an oat and flour streusel. For added fiber, vitamins, and minerals, this crumble is topped with a whole wheat flour streusel.*

YIELD: 8-inch square crumble      SERVINGS: 9
SERVING SIZE: 2⅔-inch square

| | WEIGHT | MEASURE |
|---|---|---|
| ⅛-inch thick slices peeled ripe peaches | 18 oz | 3 c (1½ pt) |
| Fresh or frozen unsweetened blackberries | 8 oz | 1⅔ c |
| Maple syrup, divided | 7 oz | ½ c + 2 tbsp |
| Cornstarch | 1½ oz | ¼ c + 1 tbsp |
| Vanilla extract | | ½ tsp |
| Whole wheat flour | 3 oz | ⅔ c |
| All-purpose flour | 2 oz | ¼ c + 3 tbsp |
| Firmly packed light brown sugar | 3 oz | ¼ c + 2 tbsp |
| Stick margarine, chilled | 1½ oz | 3 tbsp |

Preheat oven to 400 degrees F.

To peel peaches, blanch them in boiling water for 20 to 60 seconds and then place them in ice water or under cold running water until completely cooled. The skins should slip off easily. Or use thinly sliced frozen, unsweetened peaches, if desired.

Combine peaches, blackberries, 6 ounces (½ cup plus ½ tablespoon) maple syrup, cornstarch, and vanilla in a bowl. Mix together. Spoon into an 8-inch square baking pan.

Combine flours, light brown sugar, margarine, and remaining 1 ounce (1½ tablespoons) maple syrup in a medium bowl. Mix together with a pastry blender or your fingertips until crumbly. Sprinkle over fruit mixture.

Bake until topping is golden brown, or about 35 minutes. Cut into 9 squares. Serve warm, at room temperature, or chilled. Top with a scoop of vanilla fat-free frozen yogurt or a dollop of low-fat sour cream lightly sweetened with brown sugar, if desired.

---

### NUTRITIONAL FACTS

Calories: 227 (11% from fat)

Fat 3 g (.6 g sat, 1.2 g mono, 1 g poly)

Protein: 2.6 g and 4%

Carbohydrate: 49.6 g and 84%

Fiber: 3.8 g

Cholesterol: 0 mg

Iron: 1.3 mg

Sodium: 36.4 mg

Calcium: 38.9 mg

Diabetic Exchanges: 1 Starch; 1 Other Carbohydrate; 1 Fruit; ½ Fat

---

# Peanut Butter and Jelly Apple Rings Topped with Meringue

*We all know that peanut butter is packed with protein. If you are avoiding this recipe because of rumors that peanut butter is high in trans fats, reconsider. The* UC Berkeley Wellness Letter *reported that analysis by a USDA researcher found that commercial peanut butter contains virtually no trans fat. The fat in peanut butter is highly monounsaturated and this type does not raise blood cholesterol. In fact, research suggests that a diet rich in peanuts and peanut butter could significantly reduce blood cholesterol. If you are trying to eat more soy foods or are allergic to peanuts, roasted soy nut butter works well in this recipe, too.*

YIELD: 8 apple rings          SERVING SIZE: 1 apple ring

| | WEIGHT | MEASURE |
|---|---|---|
| Butter-flavored vegetable oil cooking spray | — | — |
| Golden Delicious apples, peeled and cored | 15 oz | 2 large |
| Apple juice | | 1½ c |
| Crunchy peanut butter or roasted soy nut butter | | 2 ⅔ tbsp (8 tsp) |
| 100%-fruit strawberry spread, lightly whipped, divided | | 8 tsp + ¼ c |
| Large egg white, at room temperature | 1¼ oz | 1 |

Preheat oven to 400 degrees F. Coat a baking sheet with cooking spray.

Slice each apple into 4 rings. Heat apple juice over medium heat in a large straight-sided skillet until boiling. Add apple rings. Simmer until apples are just tender, or about 5 minutes, turning once. Remove to paper towels; pat dry. Reserve apple juice for another use.

Spread each apple ring first with 1 teaspoon peanut butter and then with 1 teaspoon strawberry spread.

Place rings with strawberry spread side up on prepared baking sheet.

Using an electric mixer, beat egg white in a small mixing bowl until stiff peaks form. Fold in remaining ¼ cup strawberry spread until blended. Spoon meringue on top of apple slices, covering completely. Bake until golden brown, or about 8 minutes. Place on 8 dessert plates and serve immediately.

---

### NUTRITIONAL FACTS

| | | |
|---|---|---|
| Calories: 117 (20% from fat) | Carbohydrate: 22.5 g and 73% | Sodium: 36.6 mg |
| Fat: 2.8 g (.6 g sat, 1.3 g mono, .8 g poly) | Fiber: 2 g | Calcium: 5.7 mg |
| Protein: 1.9 g and 6% | Cholesterol: 0 mg | Diabetic Exchanges: ½ Other Carbohydrate; 1 |
| | Iron: .4 mg | Fruit; ½ Fat |

---

# Purple Plum Blueberry Oat Crunch

*Fruit crunches, crisps, and crumbles have all the charm of pies but require half the work. In this recipe, cubes of purple plums and blueberries are baked sprinkled with a crunchy streusel. Rather than lots of butter or margarine, this high-fiber rolled oat, whole wheat flour and brown sugar topping is flavored and held together with maple syrup.*

YIELD: 8-inch square crunch

SERVING SIZE: 2⅔-inch square

SERVINGS: 9

| | WEIGHT | MEASURE |
|---|---|---|
| Fresh ripe purple plums, pitted and cut into 1-inch cubes | 22 oz as purchased | 15 to 18 |
| Fresh or frozen unsweetened blueberries | 14 oz | 2¾ c (1⅜ pt) |
| Maple syrup, divided | 11 oz | 1 c |
| Firmly packed, light brown sugar, divided | 3½ oz | 3 tbsp + ¼ c |
| Instant tapioca | 1 oz | 3 tbsp |
| Finely grated orange zest | | 1 tsp |
| Long-cooking ("old-fashioned") rolled oats | 5 oz | 1⅔ c |
| Whole wheat flour | 1 oz | ¼ c |
| Stick margarine, chilled | ½ oz | 1 tbsp |
| Ground cinnamon | | 1 tsp |
| Ground ginger | | 1 tsp |
| Ground nutmeg | | ½ tsp |

Preheat oven to 350 degrees F.

Combine plums, blueberries, 8 ounces (¾ cup) maple syrup, 1½ ounces (3 tablespoons) brown sugar, tapioca, and orange zest in an 8-inch square baking pan. Toss until well mixed.

Combine remaining 2 ounces (¼ cup) brown sugar and 3 ounces (¼ cup) maple syrup, oats, flour, margarine, cinnamon, ginger, and nutmeg in a medium bowl. Mix together with a pastry blender or your fingertips until crumbly. Sprinkle crumbs over fruit mixture. Bake until fruit is tender, or about 1 hour. If top is becoming too brown, cover loosely with foil and continue baking. Cut into 9 squares. Serve warm, at room temperature, or chilled. Top with a dollop of vanilla fat-free frozen yogurt, if desired.

---

### NUTRITIONAL FACTS

Calories: 288 (9% from fat)

Fat: 3 g (.6 g sat, 1.2 g mono, 1 g poly)

Protein: 3.7 g and 5%

Carbohydrate: 64.7 g and 86%

Fiber: 4.5 g

Cholesterol: 0 mg

Iron: 4.6 mg

Sodium: 184.4 mg

Calcium: 135.4 mg

Diabetic Exchanges: 1 Starch; 2 Other Carbohydrates; 1 Fruit; ½ Fat

---

# Rhubarb Compote Laced with Dried Cranberries

*Each spring, when the cherry red stalks of rhubarb popped up in my mother's garden, I knew it wouldn't be long before our dinner table would be blessed with a bowl of rhubarb sauce. In this version of my mother's recipe, the tart rhubarb shoots are simmered in fruit juices and enriched with dried cranberries and a pinch of cinnamon and nutmeg. Although biologically rhubarb is a vegetable, it's treated as a fruit in the kitchen. Offer this compote as a condiment sauce along with meat, fish, and poultry dishes, or serve for dessert as a novel conclusion to a meal.*

YIELD: 5 c (1¼ qt) compote          SERVINGS: 10
SERVING SIZE: ½ c compote

| | WEIGHT | MEASURE |
|---|---|---|
| 1-inch pieces of fresh or frozen unsweetened rhubarb stalks | 1½ lb | 6 c (1½ qt) |
| Water | | 1 c |
| Thawed white grape juice concentrate, undiluted | | 1 c |
| Thawed apple juice concentrate, undiluted | | ½ c |
| Sweetened dried cranberries | 3 oz | scant ⅔ c |
| Ground cinnamon | | ¼ tsp |
| Ground nutmeg | | ⅛ tsp |

Combine all ingredients in a large saucepan. Heat to boiling, then reduce heat to low. Simmer uncovered, stirring often, until rhubarb is soft, or about 15 minutes. To adjust consistency, thin with additional water or thicken by simmering. Spoon into 10 dessert dishes and serve warm, at room temperature, or chilled, or offer as a topping for vanilla reduced-fat ice cream or whole grain pancakes or waffles.

| NUTRITIONAL FACTS | | |
|---|---|---|
| Calories: 109 (3% from fat) | Carbohydrate: 26.5 g and 94% | Sodium: 14.3 mg |
| Fat: .4 g (.1 g sat, 0 g mono, .1 g poly) | Fiber: 1.9 g | Calcium: 69 mg |
| Protein: .8 g and 3% | Cholesterol: 0 mg | Diabetic Exchanges: 2 Fruits |
| | Iron: .6 mg | |

# Rum-Flavored Sour Cream Gelatin Dotted with Peaches

*The creation of this gelatin was quite by accident. It began as a German-inspired sour cream mousse. After a few mistakes, this snow-white, full-bodied gelatin hinting of rum and filled with peach bits was produced. If you feel like trying something a bit unusual, this fat-free and fruit–juice sweetened dessert earns a "healthy must try."*

YIELD: 2½ c (1¼ pt) gelatin          SERVINGS: 5
SERVING SIZE: ½ c gelatin

| | WEIGHT | MEASURE |
|---|---|---|
| Thawed white grape juice concentrate, undiluted | | ½ c |
| Unflavored gelatin | | 1 envelope (scant 1 tbsp) |
| Fat-free sour cream | 9 oz | 1 c |
| Vanilla extract | | ½ tsp |
| Rum extract | | ½ tsp |
| Peeled and pitted diced peaches | 7 oz | 1 c |

Place juice concentrate in a small saucepan. Sprinkle gelatin over. Place over low heat, stirring until dissolved. Transfer to a small bowl. Add sour cream and vanilla and rum extracts. Mix until well blended. The sour cream should have lost its chill before adding to gelatin mixture. If not, set over hot water for 2 or 3 minutes.

Rinse a 3- to 4-cup bowl or mold with cold water. Shake out excess. Pour in gelatin mixture. Refrigerate until about as thick as raw egg whites, or about 1½ hours.

To peel peaches, blanch them in boiling water for 20 to 60 seconds and then place them in ice water or under cold running water until completely cooled. The skins should slip off easily. Then fold in diced peaches. If for some reason the gelatin becomes solid before fruit is incorporated, melt it over a saucepan of simmering water and start again. Refrigerate until set, or about 3 hours. Spoon gelatin into 5 dessert dishes or dip container into very hot water for a few seconds and invert onto a serving plate. Decorate with peach slices, if desired, and serve.

### *VARIATION*

Coconut-Flavored Sour Cream Gelatin with Pineapple Tidbits: Replace rum extract with ½ teaspoon pure coconut extract and diced peaches with 1 cup drained pineapple tidbits canned in juice. Do not use fresh pineapple; it contains an enzyme that prevents gelatin from setting.

---

### NUTRITIONAL FACTS

| | | |
|---|---|---|
| Calories: 132 (1% from fat) | Carbohydrate: 26.8 g and 83% | Iron: .2 mg |
| Fat: .1 g | Alcohol: .3 g and 2% | Sodium: 44.6 mg |
| Protein: 4.9 g and 15% | Fiber: .9 g | Calcium: 70.3 mg |
| | Cholesterol: 8 mg | Diabetic Exchanges: 1½ Fruits; ½ Skim Milk |

# Sweet Tofu and Yogurt Gelatin with Strawberry Bits

*Soybeans' high-protein, low-fat, and low-carbohydrate profile make them an increasingly appealing food choice for health-conscious diners. Tofu is one of the many products created from these beans. To create this gelatin, tofu is blended with yogurt and flavored and naturally sweetened with orange and apple juice concentrates. When the tofu is partially gelled, sliced strawberries are folded in. The creamy gelatin can be served as an appetizer, salad, dessert, or healthful snack.*

YIELD: 8-inch square gelatin  SERVINGS: 9
SERVING SIZE: 2⅔-inch square

|  | WEIGHT | MEASURE |
|---|---|---|
| Water |  | ¾ c |
| Unflavored gelatin |  | 1 envelope (scant 1 tbsp) |
| Thawed apple juice concentrate, undiluted |  | ¼ c + 2 tbsp |
| Thawed orange juice concentrate, undiluted |  | ¼ c |
| Fat-free plain yogurt | 6½ oz | ¾ c |
| Firm silken tofu | 5 oz | 1¼-inch-thick slice |
| Vanilla extract |  | 1 tsp |
| Red food coloring |  | few drops (optional) |
| Hulled and thinly sliced fresh ripe strawberries | 10 oz | 2 c (1 pt) |

Place water in a small saucepan. Sprinkle gelatin over. Place over low heat, stirring until dissolved. Transfer to a medium bowl. Add apple and orange juice concentrates. Stir to mix.

Combine yogurt, tofu, vanilla, and food coloring (if using) in a blender or food processor. Blend until smooth. Mix into juice mixture. Rinse an 8-inch square baking pan with cold water. Shake out excess. Pour in gelatin mixture.

Refrigerate until about as thick as raw egg whites, or about 1½ hours. Then fold in berries. If for some reason the gelatin becomes solid before fruit is incorporated, melt it over a saucepan of simmering water and start again. Refrigerate until set, or about 3 hours. Cut into 9 squares and serve.

---

### NUTRITIONAL FACTS

Calories: 66 (9% from fat)
Fat: .6 g (.1 g sat, .1 g
   mono, .3 g poly)
Protein: 3.4 g and 20%

Carbohydrate: 12 g and
   71%
Fiber: .8 g
Cholesterol: .4 mg
Iron: .5 mg

Sodium: 26.9 mg
Calcium: 55.8 mg
Diabetic Exchanges: ½
   Fruit; ½ Skim Milk

# Cakes

Aromatic Applesauce Spice Cake Studded with Raisins

Baileys Irish Cream Chocolate Cake

Chocolate-Bottomed Banana Cake

Chocolate Roulade Filled with Raspberry Frozen Yogurt

Dried Plum Cake Flavored with Aromatic Spices

Garden Fresh Carrot Cupcakes Blossoming
with Dried Cranberries

Gingerbread Cake Laced with Fresh Ginger

Gingerbread Upside Down Cake Topped with Sliced Pears

Graham Cracker Cake Topped with Glazed Dates

Homestyle Banana Cake Enriched with Sour Cream

Hot Fudge Sundae Cake Topped with Rich Chocolate Pudding

Lemon Low-Fat Custard Sponge Cake Puff

Moist Bran Cake Sprinkled with Dried Cranberries

Old-Fashioned Carrot Pineapple Raisin Cake

Pumpkin Cake Hinting of Cinnamon, Cloves, and Ginger

Pumpkin Roulade Rolled with Cream Cheese Frosting

White Whole Wheat Angel Food Spice Cake

Whole Wheat Apricot Cake Spiked with Dried Cranberries

Whole Wheat Banana Zucchini Cake Studded
with Pineapple and Raisins

# Aromatic Applesauce Spice Cake Studded with Raisins

*We all know that fruits and vegetables are good for us. Getting most North Americans to eat the recommended five or more a day is another story. To up the count, mix fruits and vegetables into cookies, bars, quick breads, and other baked goods. It's as easy as blending applesauce, prune (dried plum) purée, and raisins into this spice cake.*

YIELD: 13-by-9-inch cake      SERVINGS: 24
SERVING SIZE: 2⅛-by-2¼-inch piece

| | WEIGHT | MEASURE |
|---|---|---|
| Butter-flavored vegetable oil cooking spray | — | — |
| Granulated sugar | 8 oz | 1 c + 2 tbsp |
| Unsweetened applesauce | 6 oz | ¾ c |
| Prune purée (page 5) or prune baby food | 4 oz | ½ c |
| Large egg whites | 2½ oz | 2 |
| Large egg | 2 oz | 1 |
| All-purpose flour | 10 oz | 2¼ c |
| Baking soda | | 1½ tsp |
| Ground cinnamon | | ½ tsp |
| Ground cloves | | ¼ tsp |
| Ground nutmeg | | ¼ tsp |
| Salt | | ¼ tsp |
| Baking powder | | ¼ tsp |
| Firmly packed raisins | 6 oz | 1 c |

Preheat oven to 350 degrees F. Coat a 13-by-9-by-2-inch baking pan with cooking spray.

Combine sugar, applesauce, prune purée, egg whites, and egg in a large mixing bowl. Beat until well blended.

Combine flour, baking soda, cinnamon, cloves, nutmeg, salt, and baking powder in a medium bowl. Mix until blended. Mix in raisins. Add dry ingredients into liquid ingredients and mix until just moist.

Spread evenly in prepared pan. Bake until a wooden pick inserted in center comes out clean, or about 30 minutes. Cool cake in pan on a wire rack. Top with Maple Powdered Sugar Frosting (page 222) or icing of choice, if desired. Cut into 24 pieces and serve.

```
┌─────────────────────────────────────────────────────────────────┐
│                     NUTRITIONAL FACTS                             │
│                                                                   │
│ Calories: 121 (3% from    Carbohydrate: 28 g and    Sodium: 116.1 mg       │
│   fat)                      90%                      Calcium: 7.5 mg        │
│ Fat: .4 g (.1 g sat, .1 g  Fiber: 1.1 g             Diabetic Exchanges: ½  │
│   mono, .1 g poly)         Cholesterol: 8.9 mg        Starch; ½ Other Carbo-│
│ Protein: 2.1 g and 7%      Iron: .9 mg                hydrate; 1 Fruit      │
└─────────────────────────────────────────────────────────────────┘
```

# Baileys Irish Cream Chocolate Cake

*This cake is not an everyday chocolate cake. It's enriched with Baileys Light Irish Cream. Like the original Baileys, Baileys Light derives its chocolate cream flavor from Irish cream and whiskey, yet contains 50 percent less fat and 33 percent fewer calories than the original.*

YIELD: 13-by-9-inch cake                              SERVINGS: 24
SERVING SIZE: 2⅛-by-2¼-inch piece

|  | WEIGHT | MEASURE |
|---|---|---|
| Butter-flavored vegetable oil cooking spray | — | — |
| Granulated sugar | 14 oz | 2 c (1 pt) |
| Strong decaffeinated coffee, hot | | 1 c |
| Low-fat buttermilk | | ¾ c |
| Prune purée (page 5) or prune baby food | 6 oz | ¾ c |
| Baileys Light Irish Cream liqueur | | ¼ c |
| Large egg whites | 2½ oz | 2 |
| All-purpose flour | 8 oz | 1¾ c |
| Unsweetened cocoa powder | 3 oz | ¾ c + 2 tbsp |
| Baking powder | | 1 tbsp |
| Salt | | ½ tsp |

Preheat oven to 350 degrees F. Coat a 13-by-9-by-2-inch baking pan with cooking spray.

Combine sugar, coffee, buttermilk, prune purée, liqueur, and egg whites in a large mixing bowl. Beat until well blended.

Combine flour, cocoa powder, baking powder, and salt in a medium bowl. Mix until blended. Mix dry ingredients into liquid ingredients until just moist.

Spread evenly in prepared pan. Bake until a wooden pick inserted in center comes out clean, or about 40 minutes. Cool cake in pan on a wire rack. Sift powdered sugar over the finished cake, spread with frosting of choice, or top with Raspberry Sauce Sweetened with Fruit Juice (page 227) or fruit sauce of choice, if desired. Cut into 24 pieces and serve.

| NUTRITIONAL FACTS | | |
|---|---|---|
| Calories: 131 (5% from fat) | Carbohydrate: 31 g and 88% | Sodium: 93.8 mg |
| Fat: .8 g (.5 g sat, .2 g mono, .1 g poly) | Fiber: 1.7 g | Calcium: 19.2 mg |
| Protein: 2.4 g and 7% | Cholesterol: 1.5 mg | Diabetic Exchanges: ½ Starch; 1 Other Carbo- |
| | Iron: 1.2 mg | hydrate; ½ Fruit |

# Chocolate-Bottomed Banana Cake

*This unique cake combines two cakes in one: a moist banana cake on top and a rich chocolate cake on the bottom. While its appearance suggests it is complicated to make, it's not. Half of the banana cake's batter is flavored with cocoa powder and the other half is not.*

YIELD: 13-by-9-inch cake

SERVING SIZE: 2⅛-by-2¼-inch piece

SERVINGS: 24

| | WEIGHT | MEASURE |
|---|---|---|
| Butter-flavored vegetable oil cooking spray | — | — |
| Granulated sugar | 8 oz | 1 c + 2 tbsp |
| Stick margarine, softened | 1 oz | 2 tbsp |
| Puréed very ripe bananas (1½ lb as purchased/4 medium) | 1 lb | 2 c (1 pt) |
| Large egg whites | 2½ oz | 2 |
| Almond extract | | 1 tsp |
| All-purpose flour | 6 oz | 1⅓ c |
| Baking powder | | 1 tsp |
| Baking soda | | 1 tsp |
| Salt | | ½ tsp |
| Unsweetened cocoa powder | 1 oz | ¼ c |

Preheat oven to 350 degrees F. Coat a 13-by-9-by-2-inch baking pan with cooking spray.

Combine sugar and margarine in a large mixing bowl. Beat until well blended. Add banana purée, egg whites, and almond extract. Mix until well blended.

Combine flour, baking powder, baking soda, and salt in a small bowl. Mix until blended. Mix dry ingredients into banana mixture until just moist.

Divide batter in half. Add cocoa powder to half of batter and mix until blended. Spread evenly in prepared pan. Spoon remaining batter over and swirl into first layer with a knife.

Bake until a wooden pick inserted in center comes out clean, or about 30 minutes. Cool cake in pan on a wire rack. Sift powdered sugar over or spread with Quick-and-Easy Chocolate Icing (page 226) or other frosting, if desired. Cut into 24 pieces and serve.

---

NUTRITIONAL FACTS

Calories: 93 (12% from fat)
Fat: 1.3 g (.3 g sat, .5 g mono, .4 g poly)
Protein: 1.5 g and 6%

Carbohydrate: 20 g and 82%
Alcohol: .1 g and 0%
Fiber: 1 g
Cholesterol: 0 mg

Iron: .6 mg
Sodium: 115.8 mg
Calcium: 4.2 mg
Diabetic Exchanges: ½ Starch; 1 Fruit

# Chocolate Roulade Filled with Raspberry Frozen Yogurt

*This chocolate whole wheat sponge cake is rolled jelly roll–style with creamy, softened raspberry frozen yogurt. It's as pretty as a picture. The rich, deep brown roll is dusted with snowy white powdered sugar and decorated with fresh red raspberries tinged with purple and fresh green mint leaves.*

YIELD: 15-by-10-inch jelly roll      SERVINGS: 10
SERVING SIZE: 1-inch-wide slice

| | WEIGHT | MEASURE |
|---|---|---|
| Butter-flavored vegetable oil cooking spray | — | — |
| Parchment paper | | 1 sheet |
| Whole wheat pastry flour or whole wheat flour | 1½ oz | ⅓ c |
| Unsweetened cocoa powder | 1 oz | ¼ c |
| Baking soda | | ¼ tsp |
| Large eggs, separated | 8 oz | 4 |
| Vanilla extract | | ½ tsp |
| Firmly packed light brown sugar, divided | 7 oz | ¾ c + 2 tbsp |
| Sifted powdered sugar | 1 oz | ¼ c |
| Raspberry low-fat frozen yogurt | 12 oz | 2 c (1 pt) |

Preheat oven to 375 degrees F. Coat a 15-by-10-inch jelly roll pan with cooking spray. Line with parchment paper, and coat paper with cooking spray.

Combine flour, cocoa, and baking soda in a small bowl. Mix until blended. Set aside.

Combine egg yolks and vanilla in a small mixing bowl. Beat on high speed with an electric mixer until thick and lemon-colored, or about 5 minutes. Gradually add 3 ounces (¼ cup + 2 tablespoons) brown sugar to egg yolks, beating on high speed until sugar is nearly dissolved.

With clean beaters, beat egg whites in a large, clean mixing bowl until foamy. Gradually add remaining 4 ounces (½ cup) brown sugar, beating until stiff peaks form.

Fold egg yolk mixture into whites. Sprinkle flour mixture over whites;

fold until just blended. Pour batter into prepared pan, spreading evenly. Bake until cake springs back when lightly touched in center, or about 12 minutes.

Loosen edges of cake from pan with a spatula. Invert immediately onto a towel liberally sprinkled with powdered sugar. Remove parchment paper from cake. Trim any crusty edges. Starting with shorter side, roll up cake in towel. Cool completely on a wire rack.

Place frozen yogurt in a medium mixing bowl. Set aside until slightly softened. Once softened, beat with an electric mixer until spreadable.

Unroll cooled cake. Remove towel. Spread softened frozen yogurt within 1 inch of edges. Roll up cake starting with one of cake's shorter sides. Place seam side down on a serving plate. Cover; freeze until firm. Present with powdered sugar sifted over and decorated with fresh raspberries and mint sprigs, if desired. Cut cake roll on diagonal into ten 1-inch slices and serve.

### NUTRITIONAL FACTS

Calories: 173 (15% from fat)
Fat: 3 g (1.2 g sat, 1 g mono, .3 g poly)
Protein: 5.2 g and 11%

Carbohydrate: 33.6 g and 74%
Fiber: 1.4 g
Cholesterol: 86.6 mg
Iron: 1.2 mg

Sodium: 74.7 mg
Calcium: 85.9 mg
Diabetic Exchanges: 1 Starch; 1 Other Carbohydrate; ½ Fat

# Dried Plum Cake Flavored with Aromatic Spices

*Dried plum (better known as prune) purée adds fruity moistness to this fragrant cake while nuggets of diced prunes contribute a chewy texture and rich taste. Nutritionally, prunes are good sources of B vitamins, iron, and potassium. They are also rich in beta-carotene and fiber.*

YIELD: 8-inch square cake          SERVINGS: 9
SERVING SIZE: 2⅔-inch square

| | WEIGHT | MEASURE |
|---|---|---|
| Butter-flavored vegetable oil cooking spray | — | — |
| Granulated sugar | 6 oz | ¾ c + 2 tbsp |
| Prune purée (page 5) or prune baby food | 3 oz | ¼ c + 2 tbsp |
| Low-fat buttermilk | | ¼ c |
| Large egg whites | 2½ oz | 2 |
| Vanilla extract | | 1 tsp |
| All-purpose flour | 6 oz | 1⅓ c |
| Baking soda | | 1 tsp |
| Ground cinnamon | | ¾ tsp |
| Salt | | ½ tsp |
| Ground cloves | | ⅛ tsp |
| Ground nutmeg | | ⅛ tsp |
| Firmly packed diced pitted prunes | 6 oz | 1 c |

Preheat oven to 350 degrees F. Coat an 8-inch square baking pan with cooking spray.

Combine sugar, prune purée, buttermilk, egg whites, and vanilla in a medium mixing bowl. Mix until well blended.

Combine flour, baking soda, cinnamon, salt, cloves, and nutmeg in a medium bowl. Mix until blended. Mix in diced prunes. Mix dry ingredients into liquid ingredients until just moist.

Spread evenly in prepared pan. Bake until a wooden pick inserted in center comes out clean, or about 30 minutes. Cool cake in pan on a wire rack or serve warm. Top with Lemon Powdered Sugar Frosting with Finely Grated Zest (page 221) or frosting of choice, if desired. Cut into 9 squares and serve.

---

### NUTRITIONAL FACTS

Calories: 218 (2% from fat)
Fat: .4 g (.1 g sat, 0 g mono, .1 g poly)
Protein: 3.7 g and 6%

Carbohydrate: 51.6 g and 91%
Fiber: 2.3 g
Cholesterol: .4 mg
Iron: 1.7 mg

Sodium: 292.1 mg
Calcium: 26.3 mg
Diabetic Exchanges: 1 Starch; 1 Other Carbohydrate; 1½ Fruits

# Garden Fresh Carrot Cupcakes Blossoming with Dried Cranberries

*Next to beets, carrots have the highest sugar content of any vegetable. This may explain why babies like this vegetable so much. Besides tasting good, carrots are packed with nutrients. They supply fiber, beta-carotene (which the body converts to vitamin A), potassium, and other nutrients. They are key to the rich flavor as well as the moist and appealing texture of these cupcakes.*

*For every day, these cupcakes are ready to eat warm out of the oven or cooled. For special occasions, spread with Whipped Light Cream Cheese Frosting (page 229) and decorate with carrot roses. To prepare the carrot roses, peel thin, even strips from a carrot. Boil the strips in a simple syrup of equal parts water and sugar until the strips are pliable, or about one minute. Tightly roll a carrot strip to create a center for the flower. Continue wrapping around the center a few times, twist the strip, continue wrapping, and finish with a twist.*

YIELD: 15 cupcakes                    SERVING SIZE: 1 cupcake

|  | WEIGHT | MEASURE |
|---|---|---|
| Butter-flavored vegetable oil cooking spray | — | — |
| Fat-free milk |  | ¾ c |
| Prune purée (page 5) or prune baby food | 4 oz | ½ c |
| Granulated sugar | 4 oz | ½ c |
| Large egg whites | 2½ oz | 2 |
| Stick margarine, melted | ½ oz | 1 tbsp |
| Vanilla extract |  | 1 tsp |
| Grated carrots | 4 oz | 1 c |
| All-purpose flour | 8 oz | 1¾ c |
| Baking powder |  | 1 tbsp |
| Ground cinnamon |  | 1 tsp |
| Ground allspice |  | ¼ tsp |
| Ground nutmeg |  | ¼ tsp |
| Ground cloves |  | ⅛ tsp |
| Firmly packed sweetened dried cranberries, coarsely chopped | 4 oz | ¾ c |

Preheat oven to 375 degrees F. Coat 15 muffin cups with cooking spray.

Combine milk, prune purée, sugar, egg whites, margarine, and vanilla in a large mixing bowl. Beat until well blended. Mix in carrots until well blended.

Combine flour, baking powder, cinnamon, allspice, nutmeg, and cloves in a medium bowl. Mix until well blended. Mix in cranberries. Mix dry ingredients into liquid ingredients until just moist.

Spoon batter into prepared muffin cups dividing evenly. Do not bake in paper-lined tins as cupcakes will stick. Bake until a wooden pick inserted in center comes out clean, or about 20 minutes. Serve warm or remove to a wire rack to cool.

---

### NUTRITIONAL FACTS

| | | |
|---|---|---|
| Calories: 130 (7% from fat) | Carbohydrate: 28 g and 85% | Sodium: 112 mg |
| Fat: 1 g (.2 g sat, .4 g mono, .3 g poly) | Fiber: 1.3 g | Calcium: 25.9 mg |
| Protein: 2.8 g and 8% | Cholesterol: .2 mg | Diabetic Exchanges: 1 Starch; ½ Fruit; 1 Vegetable |
| | Iron: 1.1 mg | |

# Gingerbread Cake Laced with Fresh Ginger

*The credit for the superb taste of this moist and fragrant cake goes to freshly grated gingerroot. The peppery, slightly sweet flavor and pungent, spicy aroma of fresh ginger is very different from that of ground ginger. For best results, purchase very hard smooth-skinned gingerroot that snaps readily into pieces. Avoid roots that look dry and wrinkled and feel light.*

YIELD: 9-inch round cake

SERVING SIZE: 1 wedge (one-ninth cake)

SERVINGS: 9

| | WEIGHT | MEASURE |
|---|---|---|
| Butter-flavored vegetable oil cooking spray | — | — |
| Whole wheat pastry flour or whole wheat flour | 4 oz | scant 1 c |
| All-purpose flour | 3 oz | ⅔ c |
| Baking soda | | 1 tsp |
| Ground cinnamon | | ½ tsp |
| Salt | | ½ tsp |
| Ground cloves | | pinch |
| Ground nutmeg | | pinch |
| Water | | ½ c + 2 tbsp |
| Light molasses | | ½ c |
| Firmly packed light brown sugar | 4 oz | ½ c |
| Prune purée (page 5) or prune baby food | 2 oz | ¼ c |
| Large egg | 2 oz | 1 |
| Stick margarine, softened | 1 oz | 2 tbsp |
| Finely minced peeled gingerroot | | 2 tbsp |

Preheat oven to 350 degrees F. Coat a 9-inch round cake pan with cooking spray.

Combine flours, baking soda, cinnamon, salt, cloves, and nutmeg in a medium bowl. Mix until well blended.

Combine water and molasses in a small bowl. (For easy cleanup, measure the molasses in a cup that has been lightly coated with vegetable cooking spray.) Mix until blended.

Combine brown sugar, prune purée, egg, margarine, and gingerroot in a medium mixing bowl. Beat until well blended.

Alternately, stir flour mixture and molasses mixture into brown sugar mixture, beginning and ending with flour mixture. Mix until just moist.

Spread evenly in prepared pan. Bake until a wooden pick inserted in center comes out clean, or about 30 minutes. Cool cake in pan on a wire rack. Sift powdered sugar over, or offer with Lemon Sauce (page 222) or sauce of choice, if desired. Cut into 9 wedges and serve.

---

### NUTRITIONAL FACTS

Calories: 226 (13% from fat)
Fat: 3.5 g (.7 g sat, 1.4 g mono, 1 g poly)
Protein: 3.6 g and 6%

Carbohydrate: 46.5 g and 80%
Fiber: 2.1 g
Cholesterol: 23.6 mg
Iron: 2.8 mg
Sodium: 322.6 mg

Calcium: 77.7 mg
Diabetic Exchanges: 1 Starch; 1½ Other Carbohydrates; ½ Fruit; ½ Fat

# Gingerbread Upside Down Cake Topped with Sliced Pears

*There's no need for a big dollop of fat- and cholesterol-filled whipped cream on this aromatic spicy cake. Rather, sliced naturally sweet pears are attractively arranged in an apple juice concentrate and brown sugar syrup and baked on the bottom of the cake. When the cake is inverted, the glazed pears become its decorative top. They add fiber, vitamins, and minerals while eliminating the need for a high-sugar, high-fat frosting.*

YIELD: 9-inch round cake      SERVINGS: 9
SERVING SIZE: 1 wedge (one-ninth cake)

| | WEIGHT | MEASURE |
|---|---|---|
| Butter-flavored vegetable oil cooking spray | — | — |
| Firmly packed light brown sugar | 2 oz | ¼ c |
| Thawed apple juice concentrate, undiluted | | 2 tbsp |
| Ripe pears, peeled, cored and sliced ⅛-inch thick | 16 oz as purchased | 3 medium |
| Prune purée (page 5) or prune baby food | 4 oz | ½ c |
| Granulated sugar | 4 oz | ½ c |
| Light molasses | | ½ c |
| Large egg whites | 2½ oz | 2 |
| All-purpose flour | 6 oz | 1⅓ c |
| Ground ginger | | 1½ tsp |
| Baking powder | | 1 tsp |
| Ground cinnamon | | 1 tsp |
| Baking soda | | ½ tsp |
| Salt | | ½ tsp |
| Ground cloves | | pinch |
| Ground nutmeg | | pinch |

Preheat oven to 350 degrees F. Coat a 9-inch round cake pan with cooking spray.

Mix brown sugar and juice concentrate in bottom of pan until well blended. Spread evenly in pan. Arrange pear slices evenly over mixture.

Combine prune purée, sugar, molasses, and egg whites in a medium mixing bowl. (For easy cleanup, measure the molasses in a cup that has been lightly coated with vegetable cooking spray.) Beat until well blended.

Combine flour, ginger, baking powder, cinnamon, baking soda, salt, cloves, and nutmeg in a small bowl. Mix until blended. Mix dry ingredients into liquid ingredients until just moist.

Spread batter evenly over pears. Bake until a wooden pick inserted in center comes out clean, or about 40 minutes. Cool in pan for about 10 minutes. Place inverted serving platter over cake; turn upside down. Let stand a few minutes before removing pan. Cut into 9 wedges and serve.

---

### NUTRITIONAL FACTS

| | | |
|---|---|---|
| Calories: 243 (1% from fat) | Carbohydrate: 58.5 g and 94% | Calcium: 88.3 mg |
| Fat: .3 g (0 g sat, .1 g mono, .1 g poly) | Fiber: 2.2 g | Diabetic Exchanges: 1 Starch; 1½ Other Carbohydrates; 1½ Fruits |
| Protein: 3.1 g and 5% | Cholesterol: 0 mg | |
| | Iron: 2.4 mg | |
| | Sodium: 268 mg | |

# Graham Cracker Cake Topped with Glazed Dates

*Unlike most cakes, this gooey, date-topped cake calls for no refined white flour. It is replaced with graham cracker crumbs. The Reverend Sylvester Graham, a health food advocate, developed the popular, wholesome graham cracker snack in the 1830s. He is also the father of the coarsely ground whole wheat, graham flour used to make the honey-sweetened crackers.*

YIELD: 13-by-9-inch cake          SERVINGS: 24
SERVING SIZE: 2⅛-by-2¼-inch piece

## CAKE

| | WEIGHT | MEASURE |
|---|---|---|
| Butter-flavored vegetable oil cooking spray | — | — |
| Granulated sugar | 4 oz | ½ c |
| Low-fat buttermilk | | 1½ c |
| Large egg whites, lightly beaten | 3¾ oz | 3 |
| Graham cracker crumbs | 14 oz | 3½ c (1¾ pt) |
| Baking soda | | 1 tbsp |

## TOPPING

| | WEIGHT | MEASURE |
|---|---|---|
| Coarsely chopped seedless dates | 14 oz | 2¾ c (1⅜ pt) |
| Granulated sugar | 8 oz | 1 c + 2 tbsp |
| Hot water | | 1 c |
| All-purpose flour | | 2 tbsp |

Preheat oven to 350 degrees F. Coat a 13-by-9-by-2-inch baking pan with cooking spray.

For the cake: Combine sugar, buttermilk, and egg whites in a large mixing bowl. Beat until well blended.

Combine graham cracker crumbs and baking soda in a medium bowl. Mix until well blended. Add cracker mixture to liquid mixture. Mix until crumbs are well moistened.

Spread evenly in prepared pan. Bake until a wooden pick inserted in center comes out clean, or about 30 minutes.

For the topping: While cake is baking, combine dates, sugar, hot water, and flour in a medium saucepan. Mix well. Cook over low heat, stirring occasionally until mixture is consistency of jam. Spoon hot date mixture gently over cake hot out of oven. Refrigerate to chill. Cut into 24 pieces and serve.

---

### NUTRITIONAL FACTS

Calories: 182 (9% from fat)

Fat: 1.9 g (.4 g sat, .7 g mono, .6 g poly)

Protein: 2.5 g and 5%

Carbohydrate: 40.4 g and 86%

Fiber: 1.7 g

Cholesterol: .9 mg

Iron: .9 mg

Sodium: 281.4 mg

Calcium: 26.8 mg

Diabetic Exchanges: 1 Starch; ½ Other Carbohydrate; 1 Fruit; ½ Fat

# Homestyle Banana Cake Enriched with Sour Cream

*Very ripe bananas are the key ingredient in this cake. To ripen bananas further after purchase, store them at room temperature. For quicker results, enclose bananas in a perforated brown paper bag. Once they reach the desired ripeness, bananas may be refrigerated for several days.*

YIELD: 8-inch square cake          SERVINGS: 9
SERVING SIZE: 2⅔-inch square

|  | WEIGHT | MEASURE |
| --- | --- | --- |
| Butter-flavored vegetable oil cooking spray | — | — |
| Granulated sugar | 6 oz | ¾ c + 2 tbsp |
| Puréed very ripe bananas (2 medium-small) | 6 oz | ¾ c |
| Fat-free sour cream | 4 oz | ½ c |
| Stick margarine, softened | 1 oz | 2 tbsp |
| Large egg white | 1¼ oz | 1 |
| Vanilla extract |  | 1 tsp |
| All-purpose flour | 5 oz | 1 c + 2 tbsp |
| Baking powder |  | ½ tsp |
| Baking soda |  | ½ tsp |
| Salt |  | ½ tsp |

Preheat oven to 350 degrees F. Coat an 8-inch square baking pan with cooking spray.

Combine sugar, bananas, sour cream, margarine, egg white, and vanilla in a medium mixing bowl. Beat until well blended.

Combine flour, baking powder, baking soda, and salt in a small bowl. Mix until well blended. Mix dry ingredients into liquid ingredients until moist.

Spread batter evenly in prepared pan. Bake until a wooden pick inserted in center comes out clean, or about 40 minutes. If top is becoming too brown after 30 minutes, cover loosely with foil and continue baking. Cool cake in pan on a wire rack. Spread with Dairy-Fresh Sour Cream Frosting (page 217), if desired. Cut into 9 squares and serve.

| NUTRITIONAL FACTS | | |
|---|---|---|
| Calories: 182 (14% from fat) | Carbohydrate: 36.9 g and 80% | Sodium: 233 mg |
| Fat: 2.8 g (.5 g sat, 1.2 g mono, .9 g poly) | Fiber: .8 g | Calcium: 5 mg |
| Protein: 3.1 g and 7% | Cholesterol: 0 mg | Diabetic Exchanges: 1 Starch; ½ Other Carbohydrate; 1 Fruit; ½ Fat |
| | Iron: .8 mg | |

# Hot Fudge Sundae Cake Topped with Rich Chocolate Pudding

*Many people believe low-fat desserts can't taste as good as rich ones. One bite of this cake and "the proof is in the pudding."*

YIELD: 9-inch round cake        SERVINGS: 9
SERVING SIZE: 1 wedge (one-ninth cake)

|  | WEIGHT | MEASURE |
|---|---|---|
| Butter-flavored vegetable oil cooking spray | — | — |
| Granulated sugar | 6 oz | ¾ c + 2 tbsp |
| Fat-free milk | | ½ c |
| Prune purée (page 5) or prune baby food | 2 oz | ¼ c |
| Vanilla extract | | 1 tsp |
| All-purpose flour | 4 oz | ¾ c + 2 tbsp |
| Unsweetened cocoa powder, divided | | 5½ tbsp |
| Baking powder | | 2 tsp |
| Salt | | ¼ tsp |
| Firmly packed light brown sugar | 6 oz | ¾ c |
| Boiling water | | 1½ c |

Preheat oven to 350 degrees F. Coat a 9-inch round cake pan with cooking spray.

Combine sugar, milk, prune purée, and vanilla in a medium mixing bowl. Beat until well blended.

Combine flour, 2 tablespoons cocoa powder, baking powder, and salt in a small bowl. Mix until blended. Mix dry ingredients into liquid ingredients until moist. Spread evenly in prepared pan.

Combine brown sugar and remaining 3½ tablespoons cocoa powder in a bowl. Mix until blended. Sprinkle over batter. Pour boiling water over batter.

Bake until cake springs back when touched lightly, or about 35 minutes. Place an inverted serving platter over cake; turn upside down. Let stand a few minutes before removing pan. Cut into 9 wedges. Spoon fudge sauce over cake and serve. Store refrigerated.

---

### NUTRITIONAL FACTS

| | | |
|---|---|---|
| Calories: 213 (3% from fat) | Carbohydrate: 51.7 g and 93% | Sodium: 170 mg |
| Fat: .7 g (.3 g sat, .2 g mono, .1 g poly) | Fiber: 1.6 g | Calcium: 41.1 mg |
| Protein: 2.6 g and 5% | Cholesterol: .2 mg | Diabetic Exchanges: 1 Starch; 2 Other Carbohydrates; ½ Fruit |
| | Iron: 1.5 mg | |

# Lemon Low-Fat Custard Sponge Cake Puff

*Chances are you learned to separate eggs by cracking the shell in half, then passing the yolk back and forth between the two shells while allowing the egg white to drop into a bowl. Or perhaps you use your hands, as I was taught to do at my first cooking job. Because both eggshells and hands are possible sources of harmful microorganisms, an egg separator or funnel is a safer option and makes the process a lot easier and less messy.*

YIELD: 8 custard puffs                    SERVING SIZE: ¾ c custard puff

|  | WEIGHT | MEASURE |
|---|---|---|
| Butter-flavored vegetable oil cooking spray | — | — |
| All-purpose flour | 2½ oz | ½ c |
| Baking powder |  | ½ tsp |
| Granulated sugar, divided | 9 oz | 1¼ c |
| Large egg yolks | 1½ oz | 2 |
| Low-fat buttermilk |  | 1½ c |
| Fresh lemon juice |  | ½ c (3 medium lemons) |
| Finely grated lemon zest |  | 2 tsp |
| Large egg whites | 5 oz | 4 |

Preheat oven to 350 degrees F. Coat eight 6-ounce ramekins or ovenproof custard cups with cooking spray.

Combine flour, baking powder, and 4½ ounces (½ cup + 2 tablespoons) sugar in a large bowl. Mix well.

Beat egg yolks in a small bowl until light. Add buttermilk, lemon juice, and zest. Mix until blended. Mix liquid ingredients into dry ingredients until blended.

Beat egg whites in a mixing bowl with an electric mixer until soft peaks form. Gradually add remaining 4½ ounces (½ cup + 2 tablespoons) sugar, beating until stiff but not dry. Fold egg-white mixture into batter.

Divide evenly among prepared ramekins. Set in a flat-bottomed deep baking or roasting pan. Pour very hot water into pan half way up sides of ramekins.

Bake until puffy and golden, or about 40 minutes. Remove from water. Cool on a wire rack. Serve warm, at room temperature, or chilled. Store refrigerated.

---

### NUTRITIONAL FACTS

Calories: 206 (9% from fat)

Fat: 2.1 g (.8 g sat, .7 g mono, .3 g poly)

Protein: 5.3 g and 10%

Carbohydrate: 42.6 g and 81%

Fiber: .4 g

Cholesterol: 69.9 mg

Iron: .7 mg

Sodium: 94.7 mg

Calcium: 65.2 mg

Diabetic Exchanges: ½ Starch; 2 Other Carbohydrates; ½ Low-Fat Milk

# Moist Bran Cake Sprinkled with Dried Cranberries

*After eating one piece of this moist and hearty homestyle cake, diners are sure to assume its nutritional profile must be incorrect. It provides more fiber than a slice of most whole wheat breads, nearly no fat and cholesterol, and more protein than found in 2 tablespoons of most peanut butters. To achieve these results, fat-free plain yogurt was substituted for the traditional butter and dried cranberries replaced the chopped nuts. The egg yolks in the original recipe were omitted and the cake's batter was enriched with bran flakes cereal.*

YIELD: 8-inch square cake

SERVINGS: 9

SERVING SIZE: 2⅔-inch square

| | WEIGHT | MEASURE |
|---|---|---|
| Butter-flavored vegetable oil cooking spray | — | — |
| Fat-free plain yogurt | 6 oz | ¾ c |
| Thawed apple juice concentrate, undiluted | | ¼ c + 2 tbsp |
| Firmly packed light brown sugar | 3 oz | ¼ c + 2 tbsp |
| Large egg white | 1¼ oz | 1 |
| All-purpose flour | 6 oz | 1⅓ c |
| Baking powder | | 1 tsp |
| Baking soda | | ½ tsp |
| Ground cinnamon | | ½ tsp |
| Salt | | ¼ tsp |
| Firmly packed sweetened dried cranberries | 3 oz | ½ c |
| Bran flakes cereal | 2 oz | 1⅓ c |

Preheat oven to 350 degrees F. Coat an 8-inch square baking pan with cooking spray.

Combine yogurt, apple juice concentrate, brown sugar, and egg white in a medium mixing bowl. Beat until blended.

Combine flour, baking powder, baking soda, cinnamon, and salt in a medium bowl. Mix until well blended. Add cranberries and bran flakes; mix until blended. Mix into yogurt mixture until blended.

Spread batter evenly in prepared pan. Bake until a wooden pick inserted in center comes out clean, or 30 to 35 minutes. Cool cake in pan on a wire rack. Coat with Orange Powdered Sugar Frosting with Finely Grated Zest (page 224), if desired. Cut into 9 squares and serve.

```
┌─────────────────────────────────────────────────────────────────────┐
│                      NUTRITIONAL FACTS                                │
│                                                                       │
│ Calories: 186 (3% from   Carbohydrate: 41.9 g and   Sodium: 265.7 mg  │
│   fat)                     88%                      Calcium: 86.6 mg   │
│ Fat: .5 g (.1 g sat, .1 g  Fiber: 2.2 g            Diabetic Exchanges: 1½ │
│   mono, .2 g poly)        Cholesterol: .3 mg          Starches; ½ Other │
│ Protein: 4.3 g and 9%     Iron: 3.1 mg               Carbohydrate; ½ Fruit │
└─────────────────────────────────────────────────────────────────────┘
```

# Old-Fashioned Carrot Pineapple Raisin Cake

*The perfect description for this cream cheese frosted, moist and tender carrot cake laced with pineapple bits and plump raisins is finger-lickin' good. For a lighter version of this high beta-carotene (which the body converts to vitamin A) dessert, omit the frosting and dust with powdered sugar.*

YIELD: 13-by-9-inch cake                                   SERVINGS: 24
SERVING SIZE: 2⅛-by-2¼-inch piece

|  | WEIGHT | MEASURE |
|---|---|---|
| Butter-flavored vegetable oil cooking spray | — | — |
| Prune purée (page 5) or prune baby food | 12 oz | 1½ c |
| Firmly packed light brown sugar | 8 oz | 1 c |
| Large egg whites | 3¾ oz | 3 |
| Grated carrots | 9 oz | 2¼ c (1⅛ pt) |
| Drained crushed pineapple, canned in juice | 8 oz | 1 c |
| Firmly packed raisins | 2 oz | ⅓ c |
| All-purpose flour | 10 oz | 2¼ c (1⅛ pt) |
| Baking soda |  | 1 tbsp |
| Ground cinnamon |  | 1½ tsp |
| Ground allspice |  | ¾ tsp |
| Salt |  | ½ tsp |
| Ground nutmeg |  | ¼ tsp |

Preheat oven to 350 degrees F. Coat a 13-by-9-by-2-inch baking pan with cooking spray.

Combine prune purée, brown sugar, and egg whites in a large mixing bowl. Beat until well blended. Mix in carrots, pineapple, and raisins until well blended.

Mix flour, baking soda, cinnamon, allspice, salt, and nutmeg in a small bowl until blended. Mix dry ingredients into liquid ingredients until just moist.

Spread evenly in prepared pan. Bake until a wooden pick inserted in center comes out clean, or about 45 minutes. Cool cake in pan on a wire rack. Sift powdered sugar over or coat with Whipped Light Cream Cheese Frosting (page 229), if desired. Cut into 24 pieces and serve.

### NUTRITIONAL FACTS

Calories: 114 (2% from fat)

Fat: .2 g (0 g sat, 0 g mono, .1 g poly)

Protein: 2.1 g and 7%

Carbohydrate: 27 g and 91%

Fiber: 1.5 g

Cholesterol: 0 mg

Iron: 1.1 mg

Sodium: 221 mg

Calcium: 20.6 mg

Diabetic Exchanges: ½ Starch; ½ Other Carbohydrate; ½ Fruit; 1 Vegetable

# Pumpkin Cake Hinting of Cinnamon, Cloves, and Ginger

*The National Cancer Institute recommends that Americans strive to eat at least five servings of fruits and vegetables a day for better health. In this recipe, both pumpkin and dried plum (prune) purées contribute flavor to this moist and tender cake along with vitamins, minerals, and fiber. At the same time, these fruit purées eliminate the need for fat.*

YIELD: 8-inch square cake

SERVING SIZE: 2⅔-inch square

SERVINGS: 9

| | WEIGHT | MEASURE |
|---|---|---|
| Butter-flavored vegetable oil cooking spray | — | — |
| Canned pumpkin | 6 oz | ⅔ c |
| Firmly packed light brown sugar | 6 oz | ¾ c |
| Prune purée (page 5) or prune baby food | 3 oz | ¼ c + 2 tbsp |
| Large egg whites | 2½ oz | 2 |
| Vanilla extract | | 1½ tsp |
| All-purpose flour | 5 oz | 1 c + 2 tbsp |
| Baking powder | | ¾ tsp |
| Baking soda | | ¾ tsp |
| Ground cinnamon | | ¾ tsp |
| Ground ginger | | ¼ tsp |
| Salt | | ¼ tsp |
| Ground cloves | | ⅛ tsp |

Preheat oven to 350 degrees F. Coat an 8-inch square baking pan with cooking spray.

Combine pumpkin, brown sugar, prune purée, egg whites, and vanilla in a medium mixing bowl. Beat until well blended.

Combine flour, baking powder, baking soda, cinnamon, ginger, salt, and cloves in a small bowl. Mix until blended. Mix dry ingredients into liquid ingredients until just moist.

Spread evenly in prepared pan. Bake until a wooden pick inserted in center comes out clean, or about 25 minutes. Cool cake in pan on a wire rack. Sift powdered sugar over or top with Whipped Light Cream Cheese Frosting (page 229), if desired. Cut into 9 squares and serve.

---

### NUTRITIONAL FACTS

Calories: 166 (1% from fat)

Fat: .2 g (0 g sat, 0 g mono, .1 g poly)

Protein: 2.8 g and 7%

Carbohydrate: 38.8 g and 92%

Fiber: 1.1 g

Cholesterol: 0 mg

Iron: 1.5 mg

Sodium: 264 mg

Calcium: 53.4 mg

Diabetic Exchanges: 1 Starch; ½ Other Carbohydrate; 1 Fruit

# Pumpkin Roulade Rolled with Cream Cheese Frosting

*To create a dessert that tastes like pumpkin pie topped with whipped cream but in the form of a cake, a whole wheat pumpkin sponge cake is rolled jelly roll–style with creamy fat-free cream cheese. Like the traditional Thanksgiving treat, this moist, low-fat sponge cake is flavored with an aromatic blend of cinnamon, ginger, allspice, and cloves.*

YIELD: 15-by-10-inch jelly roll
SERVING SIZE: 1-inch slice

SERVINGS: 10

|  | WEIGHT | MEASURE |
|---|---|---|
| Butter-flavored vegetable oil cooking spray | — | — |
| Parchment paper | | 1 sheet |
| Whole wheat pastry flour or whole wheat flour | 2 oz | ½ c |
| Baking powder | | 1 tsp |
| Ground cinnamon | | 1 tsp |
| Ground ginger | | ½ tsp |
| Ground allspice | | ¼ tsp |
| Ground cloves | | ⅛ tsp |
| Large eggs, separated | 8 oz | 4 |
| Canned pumpkin | 4 oz | scant ½ c |
| Vanilla extract | | ½ tsp |
| Firmly packed light brown sugar, divided | 7 oz | ¾ c + 2 tbsp |
| Sifted powdered sugar | 1 oz | ¼ c |
| Whipped Light Cream Cheese Frosting (page 229) | | 1 recipe |

Preheat oven to 375 degrees F. Coat a 15-by-10-inch jelly roll pan with cooking spray. Line with parchment paper. Coat paper with cooking spray.

Combine flour, baking powder, cinnamon, ginger, allspice, and cloves in a medium bowl. Mix until blended.

Combine egg yolks, pumpkin, and vanilla in a small mixing bowl. Beat with an electric mixer on high speed until thick and creamy, or about 5 minutes. Gradually add 3 ounces (¼ cup + 2 tablespoons) brown sugar to egg yolk mixture, beating on high speed until sugar is nearly dissolved.

With clean beaters, beat egg whites in a clean large mixing bowl until foamy. Gradually add remaining 4 ounces (½ cup) brown sugar, beating until stiff peaks form.

Fold egg yolk mixture into whites. Sprinkle flour mixture over whites; fold in until just blended. Pour batter into pan, spreading evenly. Bake until cake springs back when lightly touched in center, or 12 to 15 minutes.

Loosen edges of cake with a spatula. Invert immediately onto a towel sprinkled liberally with powdered sugar. Remove parchment paper from cake. Trim any crusty edges. Starting with shorter side, roll up cake in towel. Cool completely on a rack.

Unroll cooled cake. Remove towel. Spread cream cheese frosting within 1 inch of edges. Roll up cake starting with one of cake's shorter sides. Chill briefly.

Cut cake roll on diagonal into ten 1-inch slices. Present on plates dusted with powdered sugar, if desired, and serve. Store refrigerated.

---

### NUTRITIONAL FACTS

Calories: 192 (10% from fat)

Fat: 2.2 g (.7 g sat, .8 g mono, .3 g poly)

Protein: 5.8 g and 12%

Carbohydrate: 37.6 g and 78%

Fiber: .9 g

Cholesterol: 87.8 mg

Iron: 1.1 mg

Sodium: 201 mg

Calcium: 36.4 mg

Diabetic Exchanges: 1½ Starches; 1 Fruit; ½ Fat

---

# White Whole Wheat Angel Food Spice Cake

*One of the most common mistakes made when producing an angel food cake is over-beating the egg whites. The egg whites for this and other angel food cakes should be beaten until soft, not stiff, unlike when making most other meringues. Over-beating the whites causes them to become dry and makes it difficult to fold in the dry ingredients. Consequently the whites rise less during baking and tend to fall more when cooling.*

YIELD: 10-inch tube cake                    SERVINGS: 16
SERVING SIZE: 1 wedge (one-sixteenth cake)

|  | WEIGHT | MEASURE |
|---|---|---|
| Granulated sugar, divided | 9 oz | 1¼ c |
| White whole wheat flour or whole wheat pastry flour | 3 oz | ½ c |
| Cake flour or all-purpose flour | 2 oz | ½ c |
| Ground cinnamon |  | 1 tsp |
| Ground nutmeg |  | ¼ tsp |
| Ground cloves |  | ¼ tsp |
| Salt |  | ⅛ tsp |
| Large egg whites, at room temperature | 15 oz | 12 |
| Cream of tartar |  | 1 tsp |
| Lemon juice |  | 1½ tsp |

Preheat oven to 375 degrees F.

Combine 4 ounces (½ cup) sugar, flours, cinnamon, nutmeg, cloves, and salt in a sifter. Sift into a medium bowl. Set aside.

Beat egg whites in a large mixing bowl with an electric mixer until foamy. Add cream of tartar. Continue beating until whites form very soft peaks. Gradually add remaining 5 ounces (¾ cup) sugar and continue beating until whites just hold soft peaks. Add lemon juice and beat until whites hold 2-inch peaks.

Sift one-third of flour mixture over whites. After sifting, gently fold flour mixture into whites until it disappears. Repeat twice.

Spread mixture evenly in an ungreased 10-inch tube pan. Bake until top is rich golden color and cake springs back when touched lightly, or about 30 minutes. Check after 20 minutes and continue checking every 5 minutes.

Remove from oven and invert. If pan has feet, just set upside down on counter; if not, invert on a heat proof funnel or bottle neck until cake is completely cool, or about 1½ hours. Once cooled, the cake should come out of the pan. If it doesn't, run a knife around the edges to loosen. Spread with Maple Powdered Sugar Frosting (page 222). Cut with a gentle sawing motion with a serrated knife into 16 pieces and serve. It can also be served with cooked fruit spooned over, if desired.

| NUTRITIONAL FACTS | | |
|---|---|---|
| Calories: 107 (1% from fat) | Carbohydrate: 23.3 g and 86% | Sodium: 59.7 mg |
| Fat: .1 g | Fiber: .8 g | Calcium: 4.3 mg |
| Protein: 3.6 g and 13% | Cholesterol: 0 mg | Diabetic Exchanges: 1 Starch; ½ Other Carbo- |
| | Iron: .6 mg | hydrate |

# Whole Wheat Apricot Cake Spiked with Dried Cranberries

*The delicate flavor of apricots is pleasantly complemented by a dash of cinnamon and cardamom and a sprinkle of sweetened and dried ruby-red cranberries in this high-fiber cake, which is also rich in beta-carotene.*

YIELD: 9-inch round cake        SERVINGS: 9
SERVING SIZE: 1 wedge (one-ninth cake)

| | WEIGHT | MEASURE |
|---|---|---|
| Butter-flavored vegetable oil cooking spray | — | — |
| Granulated sugar, divided | 7 oz | 1 c |
| Stick margarine, softened | 1 oz | 2 tbsp |
| Puréed drained apricots, canned in juice | 12 oz | 1½ c (12–14 halves) |
| Large egg whites | 5 oz | 4 |
| Low-fat buttermilk | | ½ c |
| Whole wheat pastry flour or whole wheat flour | 8 oz | 1¾ c + 2 tbsp |
| Ground cinnamon | | 1 tbsp |
| Baking powder | | 2 tsp |
| Ground cardamom | | ¼ tsp |
| Sweetened dried cranberries | 4 oz | ¾ c |

Preheat oven to 350 degrees F. Coat a 9-inch round cake pan with cooking spray.

Combine 6 ounces (¾ cup + 2 tablespoons) sugar and margarine in a large mixing bowl. Beat until blended. Add apricot purée, egg whites, and buttermilk. Mix until well blended.

Combine flour, cinnamon, baking powder, and cardamom in a medium bowl. Mix until well blended. Mix in cranberries. Mix dry ingredients into liquid ingredients until just moist.

Spread batter evenly in prepared pan. Sprinkle remaining 1 ounce (2 tablespoons) sugar evenly over top. Bake until a wooden pick inserted in center comes out clean, or about 40 minutes. If top is becoming too brown after 30 minutes, cover loosely with foil and continue baking. Cool cake in pan on a wire rack. Cut into 9 wedges and serve.

---

### NUTRITIONAL FACTS

Calories: 265 (11% from fat)

Fat: 3.2 g (.6 g sat, 1.2 g mono, .8 g poly)

Protein: 6.2 g and 9%

Carbohydrate: 53.9 g and 80%

Fiber: 5 g

Cholesterol: .8 mg

Iron: 1.7 mg

Sodium: 124.9 mg

Calcium: 31.8 mg

Diabetic Exchanges: 2 Starches; 1 Other Carbohydrate; ½ Fruit; ½ Fat

---

# Whole Wheat Banana Zucchini Cake Studded with Pineapple and Raisins

*As the name of this moist, low-fat, low-cholesterol cake suggests, it's enriched with whole wheat flour as well as three fruits and a vegetable. Besides coming up tops in vitamins, minerals, and fiber, these goodies are what make it taste so good.*

YIELD: 13-by-9-inch cake                    SERVINGS: 24
SERVING SIZE: 2⅛-by-2¼-inch piece

| | WEIGHT | MEASURE |
|---|---|---|
| Butter-flavored vegetable oil cooking spray | — | — |
| Unpacked grated zucchini with skin | 18 oz | 3½ c (1¾ pt) |
| Salt | | ½ tsp |
| Chopped walnuts | 3 oz | ¾ c |
| Puréed very ripe bananas (4 medium) | 18 oz | 2¼ c (1⅛ pt) |
| Drained crushed pineapple, canned in juice | 12 oz | 1½ c |
| Large egg whites | 5 oz | 4 |
| Large egg | 2 oz | 1 |
| All-purpose flour | 9 oz | 2 c (1 pt) |
| Whole wheat pastry flour or whole wheat flour | 6 oz | 1⅓ c |
| Firmly packed light brown sugar | 6 oz | ¾ c |
| Baking soda | | 1⅓ tbsp |
| Ground cinnamon | | 1½ tsp |
| Ground nutmeg | | ¾ tsp |
| Ground cloves | | ¾ tsp |
| Ground allspice | | ¾ tsp |
| Firmly packed raisins | 4 oz | ⅔ c |

Preheat oven to 350 degrees F. Coat a 13-by-9-by-2-inch baking pan with cooking spray.

Place zucchini in a strainer. Sprinkle with salt. Mix to coat. Let stand for about 15 minutes. Meanwhile toast nuts by cooking in a dry nonstick skillet over medium heat, stirring constantly, until they just begin to become fragrant, or about 4 minutes. Set aside.

Squeeze zucchini with your hands to remove as much liquid as possible; discard liquid. There should be about 12 ounces (2½ cups) zucchini. Combine banana, pineapple, egg whites, egg, and zucchini in a large mixing bowl. Mix until well blended.

Combine flours, brown sugar, baking soda, cinnamon, nutmeg, cloves, and allspice in a medium bowl. Mix until well blended. Mix in raisins and walnuts. Mix dry ingredients into liquid ingredients until just moist.

Spread evenly in prepared pan. Bake until a wooden pick inserted in center comes out clean, or about 50 minutes. Cover cake loosely with foil if it is becoming too brown after 30 minutes. Cool in pan on a wire rack. Spread with Whipped Light Cream Cheese Frosting (page 229), or sift powdered sugar over, if desired. Cut into 24 pieces and serve.

## NUTRITIONAL FACTS

Calories: 163 (15% from fat)

Fat: 2.9 g (.4 g sat, .6 g mono, 1.6 g poly)

Protein: 4.1 g and 10%

Carbohydrate: 32.2 g and 75%

Fiber: 2.5 g

Cholesterol: 8.8 mg

Iron: 1.4 mg

Sodium: 304 mg

Calcium: 25.3 mg

Diabetic Exchanges: ½ Starch; 1 Other Carbohydrate; ½ Fruit; 1 Vegetable; ½ Fat

# Cookies and Bars

Applesauce Spice Cookies Dotted with Raisins

Cakelike Dark Fudge Beanie Brownies

Carrot Raisin Cookies Topped with Lemon Frosting

Chocolate Brownies Just Like Mom's

Cinnamon-Sugar Topped Sour Cream Bars
with Brandy-Plumped Raisins

Coconut-Flavored Chocolate Brownie Bars

Crispy Rice Bars Dotted with Apricot Bits

Golden Pumpkin Cookies Spiked with Date Bits

Lemon Meringue Kisses Sprinkled with Sugar Crystals

Nutty Chocolate Peanut Butter Brownies

Peanut Butter and Honey Crunch Bars

Pumpkin Pie Bars Dotted with Raisins

Soft Molasses Sour Cream Cookies

Sugar Coated Molasses Jumbles

Wholesome Apple Spice Oat Bars

# Applesauce Spice Cookies Dotted with Raisins

*Applesauce, cloves, and cinnamon taste nice combined in these cakelike, raisin-filled cookies. Top them with a swirl of creamy Maple Powdered Sugar Frosting for an "uptown" look and taste.*

YIELD: 48 cookies                    SERVING SIZE: 1 cookie

|  | WEIGHT | MEASURE |
|---|---|---|
| Butter-flavored vegetable oil cooking spray | — | — |
| Lightly packed light brown sugar | 11 oz | 1½ c |
| Unsweetened applesauce | 3 oz | ¼ c + 2 tbsp |
| Prune purée (page 5) or prune baby food | 2 oz | ¼ c |
| Large egg whites | 2½ oz | 2 |
| Vanilla extract | | 1 tsp |
| All-purpose flour | 11 oz | 2½ c (1⅛ pt) |
| Salt | | 1 tsp |
| Ground cinnamon | | 1 tsp |
| Baking soda | | ½ tsp |
| Ground cloves | | ¼ tsp |
| Firmly packed raisins | 4 oz | ⅔ c |

Preheat oven to 375 degrees F. Coat 2 or 3 baking sheets with cooking spray.

Combine brown sugar, applesauce, prune purée, egg whites, and vanilla in a large bowl. Mix until well blended.

Combine flour, salt, cinnamon, baking soda, and cloves in a medium bowl. Mix until blended. Mix in raisins. Mix dry ingredients into liquid ingredients until blended.

Drop dough by rounded teaspoonfuls onto baking sheets about 1 inch apart. Bake until almost no indentation remains when touched, or about 10 minutes. Remove immediately to a wire rack to cool. Top with Maple Powdered Sugar Frosting (page 222), if desired.

NUTRITIONAL FACTS

Calories: 58 (1% from fat)    Fiber: .4 g                Calcium: 8.8 mg
Fat: .1 g                      Cholesterol: 0 mg         Diabetic Exchanges: ½
Protein: .9 g and 6%           Iron: .5 mg                 Starch; ½ Other Carbo-
Carbohydrate: 13.8 g and       Sodium: 66.9 mg            hydrate
    93%

# Cakelike Dark Fudge Beanie Brownies

*These brownies are not related to Beanie Babies, the popular children's toys, or to the skullcaps worn by schoolchildren in the 1950s. Rather, these low-fat, cholesterol-free, nutrient-dense, dark chocolate brownies are enriched with kidney bean purée. The kidney beans add protein, fiber, vitamins, and minerals to the brownies while giving them a full-fat mouthfeel.*

YIELD: 13-by-9-inch brownies                    SERVINGS: 24
SERVING SIZE: 2⅛-by-2¼-inch piece

|  | WEIGHT | MEASURE |
|---|---|---|
| Butter-flavored vegetable oil cooking spray | — | — |
| Canned, unseasoned kidney beans (not drained) | 15¼ oz | |
| Large egg whites, divided | 12½ oz | 10 |
| Sugar | 15 oz | 2 c (1 pt) |
| Unsweetened cocoa powder | 2½ oz | ¾ c |
| All-purpose flour | 2 oz | ¼ c + 3 tbsp |
| Chopped walnuts | 1 oz | ¼ c |
| Stick margarine, melted | ½ oz | 1 tbsp |

Preheat oven to 350 degrees F. Coat a 13-by-9-by-2-inch pan with cooking spray.

Place beans in a strainer; rinse under cold water and drain well. Combine drained beans and 2 egg whites (2½ ounces) in a blender or food processor. Blend until smooth. Add remaining egg whites. Blend until mixed.

Combine sugar, cocoa, and flour in a bowl. Mix until blended. Mix in nuts. Add bean mixture and melted margarine to dry ingredients. Mix until blended.

Spread evenly in prepared pan. Bake until brownies begin to pull away from sides of the pan, or about 35 to 40 minutes. Cool in pan on a wire rack. Cut into 24 bars and serve.

| NUTRITIONAL FACTS | | |
|---|---|---|
| Calories: 113 (12% from fat) | Carbohydrate: 23.3 g and 77% | Sodium: 75.7 mg |
| | | Calcium: 9.6 mg |
| Fat: 1.6 g (.4 g sat, .5 g mono, .6 g poly) | Fiber: 1.6 g | Diabetic Exchanges: ½ Starch; 1 Other Carbo- |
| Protein: 3.3 g and 11% | Cholesterol: 0 mg | hydrate; ½ Fat |
| | Iron: .7 mg | |

# Carrot Raisin Cookies Topped with Lemon Frosting

*There's no need to limit carrots to vegetable side dishes, soups, salads, and the occasional cake. You can feature this popular year-round root vegetable, rich in beta-carotene, in all your favorite sweets—cookies, bars, muffins, quick breads, pancakes, puddings, frozen yogurts, and even pies. For best results, select firm, young, slender carrots that are free of cracks and without deep discoloration around their stems.*

YIELD: 42 cookies                    SERVING SIZE: 1 cookie

| | WEIGHT | MEASURE |
|---|---|---|
| Butter-flavored vegetable oil cooking spray | — | — |
| Unpacked light brown sugar | 7 oz | 1⅓ c |
| Prune purée (page 5) or prune baby food | 2 oz | ¼ c |
| Unsweetened applesauce | 2 oz | ¼ c |
| Large egg white | 1¼ oz | 1 |
| All-purpose flour | 10 oz | 2¼ c (1⅛ pt) |
| Grated carrots | 6 oz | 1½ c |
| Firmly packed raisins | 3 oz | ½ c |
| Chopped walnuts, toasted without fat | 2 oz | ½ c |
| Baking powder | | 2 tsp |
| Finely grated lemon zest | | 2 tsp |
| Ground nutmeg | | ½ tsp |
| Salt | | ¼ tsp |
| Lemon Powdered Sugar Frosting with Finely Grated Zest (page 221) | | 1 recipe |

Preheat oven to 375 degrees F. Coat 2 or 3 baking sheets with cooking spray.

Combine brown sugar, prune purée, applesauce, and egg white in a large bowl. Mix until well blended. Add flour, carrots, raisins, walnuts, baking powder, lemon zest, nutmeg, and salt. Mix until blended.

Drop dough by round teaspoonfuls onto prepared baking sheets about 2 inches apart. Bake until almost no indentation remains when touched, or about 12 minutes. Remove immediately to a wire rack to cool. Top with Lemon Powdered Sugar Frosting.

---

### NUTRITIONAL FACTS

Calories: 79 (10% from fat)

Fat: .9 g (.1 g sat, .2 g mono, .5 g poly)

Protein: 1.2 g and 6%

Carbohydrate: 17.1 g and 84%

Fiber: .6 g

Cholesterol: 0 mg

Iron: .6 mg

Sodium: 30.5 mg

Calcium: 8.3 mg

Diabetic Exchanges: ½ Starch; ½ Other Carbohydrate

# Chocolate Brownies
# Just Like Mom's

*You can indulge yourself with these rich and cakelike, low-fat chocolate brownies without much concern for fat or calories. One serving adds less than 1 gram of fat and a mere 89 calories. Dust with powdered sugar, and moms everywhere will feel proud to lend their name to these treats.*

YIELD: 13-by-9-inch brownies          SERVINGS: 24
SERVING SIZE: 2½-by-2¼-inch piece

|  | WEIGHT | MEASURE |
|---|---|---|
| Butter-flavored vegetable oil cooking spray | — | — |
| Prune purée (page 5) or prune baby food | 5 oz | ½ c + 2 tbsp |
| Light corn syrup | 4 oz | ⅓ c |
| Fat-free milk |  | ½ c |
| Vanilla extract |  | ½ tsp |
| Granulated sugar | 6 oz | ¾ c + 2 tbsp |
| Large egg whites | 2½ oz | 2 |
| Large egg | 2 oz | 1 |
| All-purpose flour | 5 oz | 1 c + 2 tbsp |
| Unsweetened cocoa powder | 2 oz | ½ c + 1 tbsp |
| Baking powder |  | 1 tsp |
| Salt |  | ½ tsp |
| Baking soda |  | ¼ tsp |

Preheat oven to 325 degrees F. Coat a 13-by-9-by-2-inch baking pan with cooking spray.

Combine prune purée, corn syrup, milk, and vanilla in a small bowl. Mix until well blended.

Combine sugar, egg whites, and egg in a large bowl. Beat until thick but not stiff. Add prune mixture and mix until well blended.

Combine flour, cocoa, baking powder, salt, and baking soda in a small bowl. Mix until blended. Mix dry ingredients into liquid ingredients until blended.

Spread evenly in prepared pan. Bake until a wooden pick inserted in center comes out clean, or about 24 minutes. Cool in pan on a wire rack. Sift powdered sugar over brownies, if desired. Cut into 24 bars and serve.

## NUTRITIONAL FACTS

Calories: 89 (6% from fat)

Fat: .6 g (.3 g sat, .2 g mono, .1 g poly)

Protein: 1.9 g and 8%

Carbohydrate: 20.7 g and 86%

Fiber: 1.1 g

Cholesterol: 9 mg

Iron: .8 mg

Sodium: 88.8 mg

Calcium: 13.5 mg

Diabetic Exchanges: ½ Starch; ½ Other Carbohydrate; ½ Fruit

# Cinnamon-Sugar Topped Sour Cream Bars with Brandy-Plumped Raisins

*If you like to sprinkle cinnamon sugar on your morning toast, you are sure to like these bars. A combination of puréed cooked sweet potatoes and fat-free sour cream keeps the bars moist while reducing their fat content and enhancing their nutritional value.*

YIELD: 13-by-9-inch bars

SERVING SIZE: 2⅛-by-2¼-inch piece

SERVINGS: 24

|  | WEIGHT | MEASURE |
|---|---|---|
| Butter-flavored vegetable oil cooking spray | — | — |
| Firmly packed raisins | 2 oz | ⅓ c |
| Brandy | | 2 tbsp |
| Firmly packed light brown sugar, divided | 7 oz | ¾ c + 2 tbsp |
| Mashed, peeled sweet potatoes, cooked without salt, or canned drained and mashed sweet potatoes | 6 oz | ¾ c |
| Fat-free sour cream | 3 oz | ⅓ c |
| Stick margarine, softened | 1 oz | 2 tbsp |
| Large egg white | 1¼ oz | 1 |
| Vanilla extract | | 1 tsp |
| All-purpose flour | 5 oz | 1 c + 2 tbsp |
| Baking powder | | ½ tsp |
| Baking soda | | ½ tsp |
| Salt | | ¼ tsp |
| Ground cinnamon | | 2 tsp |

Preheat oven to 350 degrees F. Coat a 13-by-9-by-2-inch baking pan with cooking spray.

Combine raisins and brandy in a small saucepan. Heat to a boil, then remove from heat and set aside to let raisins plump in brandy.

Combine 6 ounces (¾ cup) brown sugar, sweet potatoes, sour cream, margarine, egg white, and vanilla in a large bowl. Mix until well blended.

Combine flour, baking powder, baking soda, and salt in a small bowl. Mix until well blended. Mix in raisins. Mix dry ingredients into liquid ingredients until blended. Spread batter evenly in prepared pan.

Combine cinnamon and remaining 1 ounce (2 tablespoons) brown sugar in a small bowl. Mix until well blended.

Sprinkle mixture evenly over bars. Bake until a wooden pick inserted in center comes out clean, or about 20 minutes. Cool in pan on a wire rack. Cut into 24 bars and serve.

---

### NUTRITIONAL FACTS

Calories: 82 (11% from fat)
Fat: 1 g (.2 g sat, .4 g mono, .3 g poly)
Protein: 1.2 g and 6%

Carbohydrate: 16.8 g and 80%
Alcohol: .3 g and 3%
Fiber: .5 g
Cholesterol: 0 mg
Iron: .6 mg

Sodium: 78.9 mg
Calcium: 17.9 mg
Diabetic Exchanges: ½ Starch; ½ Other Carbohydrate

# Coconut-Flavored Chocolate Brownie Bars

*Most nuts are concentrated sources of fat and calories. Coconut is no exception. Fresh coconut derives 85 percent of its calories from fat. These bars are prepared with a combination of toasted and flaked sweetened coconut and pure coconut extract. The result is less fat and calories without sacrificing coconut's rich, tropical flavor. Pure coconut extract is a must—some imitation coconut extracts smell like suntan lotion. To toast flaked coconut, cook it in a nonstick skillet over medium heat, stirring constantly until golden brown. Because coconut is naturally high in fat, there's no need to coat the pan with oil before toasting.*

YIELD: 13-by-9-inch bars                SERVINGS: 24
SERVING SIZE: 2⅛-by-2¼-inch piece

| | WEIGHT | MEASURE |
| --- | --- | --- |
| Butter-flavored vegetable oil cooking spray | — | — |
| Unsweetened applesauce | 8 oz | 1 c |
| Firmly packed light brown sugar | 6 oz | ¾ c |
| Large egg whites | 5 oz | 4 |
| Pure coconut extract | | 2 tsp |
| All-purpose flour | 5 oz | 1 c + 2 tbsp |
| Flaked sweetened coconut, toasted without oil | 2 oz | ¾ c |
| Unsweetened cocoa powder | 2 oz | ½ c + 1 tbsp |
| Baking powder | | 2 tsp |
| Salt | | ½ tsp |

Preheat oven to 350 degrees F. Coat a 13-by-9-by-2-inch baking pan with cooking spray.

Combine applesauce, brown sugar, egg whites, and coconut extract in a large bowl. Mix until well blended.

Combine flour, coconut, cocoa powder, baking powder, and salt in a medium bowl. Mix until well blended. Mix dry ingredients into liquid ingredients until blended.

Spread batter evenly in prepared pan. Bake until a wooden pick inserted in center comes out clean, about 20 minutes. Cool in pan on a wire rack. Sift powdered sugar over or coat with Cocoa Mocha Frosting (page 215), if desired. Cut into 24 bars and serve.

```
┌─────────────────────────────────────────────────────────────────────┐
│                        NUTRITIONAL FACTS                              │
│                                                                       │
│  Calories: 73 (14% from      Carbohydrate: 15.1 g and   Sodium: 108 mg│
│    fat)                        76%                      Calcium: 33.5 mg│
│  Fat: 1.2 g (.9 g sat, .2 g  Alcohol: .1 g and 1%      Diabetic Exchanges: ½│
│    mono, .1 g poly)          Fiber: 1.2 g                Starch; ½ Other Carbo-│
│  Protein: 1.7 g and 9%       Cholesterol: 0 mg          hydrate       │
│                              Iron: .8 mg                              │
└─────────────────────────────────────────────────────────────────────┘
```

# Crispy Rice Bars Dotted with Apricot Bits

*All-time favorite marshmallow-coated crispy rice treats are hard to beat. For an updated fat- and cholesterol-free version that is vitamin- and mineral-rich, omit the butter or margarine and add a swirl of apricot spread and a sprinkle of apricot bits.*

YIELD: 8-inch square bars                       SERVINGS: 9
SERVING SIZE: 2⅔-inch square

|  | WEIGHT | MEASURE |
|---|---|---|
| Butter-flavored vegetable oil cooking spray | — | — |
| Miniature marshmallows | 5 oz | 2½ c (1¼ pt) |
| 100%-fruit apricot spread | 2 oz | 3 tbsp |
| Oven-toasted rice cereal | 3½ oz | 3½ c (1¾ pt) |
| Dried apricot bits | 2 oz | ⅓ c |

Coat an 8-inch square baking pan with cooking spray.

Combine marshmallows and apricot spread in a large saucepan. Cook over low heat, stirring until completely melted. Remove from heat.

Stir in cereal and apricot bits until well mixed. Use a piece of wax paper or the back of a spoon coated with cooking spray to pat mixture evenly in prepared pan. When cool, cut into 9 squares and serve.

NUTRITIONAL FACTS

| | | |
|---|---|---|
| Calories: 123 (1% from fat) | Carbohydrate: 29.9 g and 95% | Sodium: 127.1 mg |
| Fat: .2 g (.1 g sat, 0 g mono, .1 g poly) | Fiber: .5 g | Calcium: 4.7 mg |
| Protein: 1.3 g and 4% | Cholesterol: 0 mg | Diabetic Exchanges: ½ Starch; 1 Other Carbo- |
| | Iron: .9 mg | hydrate; ½ Fruit |

# Golden Pumpkin Cookies Spiked with Date Bits

*For diners who want a little taste of something sweet at the end of a meal, these bite-size, beta carotene–rich pumpkin drop cookies are just the thing. To prevent their bottoms from burning, bake these and other cookies on two baking sheets stacked together.*

YIELD: 48 cookies          SERVING SIZE: 1 cookie

| | WEIGHT | MEASURE |
|---|---|---|
| Butter-flavored vegetable oil cooking spray | — | — |
| Canned pumpkin | 12 oz | 1⅓ c |
| Granulated sugar | 8 oz | 1 c + 2 tbsp |
| Large egg whites | 2½ oz | 2 |
| All-purpose flour | 8 oz | 1¾ c |
| Baking powder | | 1 tsp |
| Baking soda | | 1 tsp |
| Ground cinnamon | | 1 tsp |
| Ground nutmeg | | ¼ tsp |
| Salt | | ¼ tsp |
| Ground ginger | | ⅛ tsp |
| Diced seedless dates | 7 oz | 1¼ c |

Preheat oven to 325 degrees F. Coat 2 or 3 baking sheets with cooking spray.

Combine pumpkin, sugar, and egg whites in a large bowl. Mix until well blended.

Combine flour, baking powder, baking soda, cinnamon, nutmeg, salt, and ginger in a medium bowl. Mix until blended. Mix in dates. Mix dry ingredients into liquid ingredients until blended.

Drop dough by rounded teaspoonfuls onto prepared baking sheets about 1 inch apart. Bake until almost no indentation remains when touched, or about 18 minutes. Remove immediately to a wire rack to cool. Top with Orange Powdered Sugar Frosting with Finely Grated Zest (page 224), if desired, and serve.

---

### NUTRITIONAL FACTS

Calories: 55 (1% from fat)   Fiber: .5 g   Calcium: 5.4 mg
Fat: .1 g   Cholesterol: 0 mg   Diabetic Exchanges: ½
Protein: .8 g and 6%   Iron: .4 mg   Other Carbohydrate; ½
Carbohydrate: 13.3 g and   Sodium: 54.4 mg   Fruit
    93%

---

# Lemon Meringue Kisses Sprinkled with Sugar Crystals

*This recipe calls for egg whites at room temperature. The proteins in eggs are more elastic when warmer. Traditionally, the temperature of eggs was raised by removing them from the refrigerator and then holding them at room temperature for several hours or until use. To prevent foodborne illness, this method is now discouraged. Temperatures between 40 and 140 degrees F are considered an ideal range for harmful bacteria to grow. A better method to raise the temperature of raw eggs quickly is to place whole unshelled eggs in a bowl of warm water or hold them under a stream of warm water until they reach room temperature.*

YIELD: 24 kisses

SERVING SIZE: 1 kiss

| | WEIGHT | MEASURE |
|---|---|---|
| Parchment paper | | 2 sheets |
| Large egg whites, at room temperature | 2½ oz | 2 |
| Yellow food coloring | | 2 drops (optional) |
| Cream of tartar | | ⅛ tsp |
| Salt | | pinch |
| Granulated sugar | 2½ oz | ⅓ c |
| Lemon extract | | 1 tsp |
| Yellow sparkling sugar crystals | ½ oz | 1 tbsp |

Preheat oven to 250 degrees F. Line 2 baking sheets with parchment paper.

Combine egg whites and food coloring (if using) in a medium mixing bowl. Beat with an electric mixer until foamy. Add cream of tartar and salt. Continue beating egg whites until thick and glossy. Add sugar gradually, continuing to beat until stiff peaks form. Fold in lemon extract.

Drop meringue by tablespoonfuls onto lined baking sheets. Sprinkle with sparkling sugar crystals. Bake 1 hour. Turn oven off and let kisses cool in unopened oven (don't look!) for 1½ to 2 hours, then serve.

## *VARIATIONS*

Replace the yellow food coloring, lemon extract, and yellow sparkling crystals as follows:

- Licorice Meringue Kisses: no food coloring, 1 teaspoon anise extract, blue sparkling sugar crystals
- Strawberry Meringue Kisses: 4 drops red food coloring (optional), 1½ teaspoons strawberry extract, red sparkling sugar crystals

---

### NUTRITIONAL FACTS

| | | |
|---|---|---|
| Calories: 15 (0% from fat) | Alcohol: .03 g and 1% | Sodium: 10.7 mg |
| Fat: 0 g | Fiber: 0 g | Calcium: .2 mg |
| Protein: .3 g and 7% | Cholesterol: 0 mg | Diabetic Exchanges: Free |
| Carbohydrate: 3.6 g and 91% | Iron: 0 mg | Food |

# Nutty Chocolate Peanut Butter Brownies

*Two ingredients that naturally go together are combined in these moist cakelike brownies: chocolate and peanut butter. Make the peanut butter chunky for the crunchy texture its bits of toasted nuts add to these bars.*

YIELD: 13-by-9-inch brownies

SERVING SIZE: 2⅛-by-2¼-inch piece

SERVINGS: 24

| | WEIGHT | MEASURE |
|---|---|---|
| Butter-flavored vegetable oil cooking spray | — | — |
| Prune purée (page 5) or prune baby food | 6 oz | ¾ c |
| Light corn syrup | 4 oz | ⅓ c |
| Chunky peanut butter | 4 oz | ½ c |
| Fat-free milk | | ¼ c |
| Vanilla extract | | ½ tsp |
| Large egg whites | 6¼ oz | 5 |
| Granulated sugar | 6 oz | ¾ c + 2 tbsp |
| All-purpose flour | 4 oz | ¾ c + 2 tbsp |
| Unsweetened cocoa powder | 2½ oz | ¾ c |
| Baking powder | | 1 tsp |
| Baking soda | | ½ tsp |
| Salt | | ¼ tsp |

Preheat oven to 325 degrees F. Coat a 13-by-9-by-2-inch baking pan with cooking spray.

Combine prune purée, corn syrup, peanut butter, milk, and vanilla in a medium bowl. Mix until well blended.

Combine egg whites and sugar in a large mixing bowl. Beat with an electric mixer until thick but not stiff. Add prune mixture and mix until well blended.

Combine flour, cocoa, baking powder, baking soda, and salt in a small bowl. Mix until well blended. Mix dry ingredients into liquid ingredients until blended.

Spread evenly in prepared pan. Bake until a wooden pick inserted in center comes out clean, or about 30 minutes. Cool in pan on a wire rack. Sift powdered sugar over or spread with frosting of choice, if desired. Cut into 24 bars and serve.

## NUTRITIONAL FACTS

Calories: 106 (23% from fat)

Fat: 2.9 g (.6 g sat, 1.4 g mono, .8 g poly)

Protein: 3.1 g and 11%

Carbohydrate: 19.3 g and 67%

Fiber: 1.6 g

Cholesterol: 0 mg

Iron: .8 mg

Sodium: 76.7 mg

Calcium: 12.5 mg

Diabetic Exchanges: ½ Starch; ½ Other Carbohydrate; ½ Fruit; ½ Fat

# Peanut Butter and Honey Crunch Bars

*Coat crackling grains of crispy rice cereal, crispy flakes of toasted rice cereal, crunchy nuggets of natural wheat and barley cereal, and soft and sweet dried apricot bits with a mixture of melted marshmallows, peanut butter, and honey; pat mixture in a pan and these treats are ready to eat. Offer as an on-the-go breakfast bar, mid-morning or afternoon pick-me-up snack, or sweet conclusion to a midday or an evening meal.*

YIELD: 13-by-9-inch bars

SERVING SIZE: 2⅛-by-2¼-inch piece

SERVINGS: 24

| | WEIGHT | MEASURE |
|---|---|---|
| Butter-flavored vegetable oil cooking spray | — | — |
| Dried apricot bits | 5 oz | 1 c |
| Miniature marshmallows | 5 oz | 2½ c (1¼ pt) |
| Chunky peanut butter | 4 oz | ½ c |
| Honey | 4 oz | ⅓ c |
| Oven-toasted rice cereal | 3 oz | 3 c (1½ pt) |
| Lightly toasted rice cereal | 3 oz | 3 c (1½ pt) |
| Natural wheat and barley cereal | 3 oz | ¾ c |

Coat a 13-by-9-by-2-inch baking pan with cooking spray.

Combine apricots, marshmallows, peanut butter, and honey in a large saucepan. Cook over low heat, stirring, until marshmallows are melted.

Remove mixture from heat. When cool, mix in cereals. Spread evenly in prepared pan. Refrigerate until firm. Cut into 24 bars and serve.

---

### NUTRITIONAL FACTS

Calories: 116 (18% from fat)

Fat: 2.5 g (.5 g sat, 1.1 g mono, .7 g poly)

Protein: 2.9 g and 9%

Carbohydrate: 22 g and 72%

Fiber: 1.1 g

Cholesterol: 0 mg

Iron: 2.5 mg

Sodium: 117.3 mg

Calcium: 6.5 mg

Diabetic Exchanges: ½ Starch; ½ Other Carbohydrate; ½ Fruit; ½ Fat

---

# Pumpkin Pie Bars Dotted with Raisins

*Pumpkin has been popular in pie since colonial times, but the sweet, beta-carotene-rich gourd is equally delicious in these moist bars. While often considered to be a vegetable, this winter squash is actually a fruit.*

YIELD: 13-by-9-inch bars

SERVINGS: 24

SERVING SIZE: 2⅛-by-2¼-inch piece

|  | WEIGHT | MEASURE |
|---|---|---|
| Butter-flavored vegetable oil cooking spray | — | — |
| Large egg whites | 7½ oz | 6 |
| Firmly packed light brown sugar | 13 oz | 1⅔ c |
| Canned pumpkin | 1 lb | 1¾ c |
| Firmly packed raisins | 4 oz | ⅔ c |
| Stick margarine, melted | 1 oz | 2 tbsp |
| All-purpose flour | 8 oz | 1¾ c |
| Baking powder |  | 2 tsp |
| Ground cinnamon |  | 1 tsp |
| Ground ginger |  | ½ tsp |
| Salt |  | ½ tsp |
| Ground allspice |  | ¼ tsp |
| Ground cloves |  | ⅛ tsp |

Preheat oven to 350 degrees F. Coat a 13-by-9-by-2-inch baking pan with cooking spray.

Place egg whites in a large mixing bowl. Beat with an electric mixer until frothy. Gradually add brown sugar, beating until well blended. Add pumpkin, raisins, and margarine. Beat until well mixed.

Combine flour, baking powder, cinnamon, ginger, salt, allspice, and cloves in a small bowl. Mix until blended. Fold dry ingredients into egg mixture until just blended.

Spread evenly in prepared pan. Bake until a wooden pick inserted in center comes out clean, or about 35 minutes. Cool in pan on a wire rack. Sift powdered sugar over, if desired. Cut into 24 pieces and serve, perhaps with a dollop of vanilla fat-free frozen yogurt.

---

### NUTRITIONAL FACTS

Calories: 139 (7% from fat)

Fat: 1.1 g (.2 g sat, .5 g mono, .4 g poly)

Protein: 2.2 g and 6%

Carbohydrate: 31.1 g and 87%

Fiber: .6 g

Cholesterol: 0 mg

Iron: 1.1 mg

Sodium: 151 mg

Calcium: 26.1 mg

Diabetic Exchanges: ½ Starch; 1 Other Carbohydrate; ½ Fruit

---

# Soft Molasses Sour Cream Cookies

*These cookies obtain their distinct flavor from light molasses, which is richer in iron, calcium, and potassium than white granulated sugar. While the light molasses used in these cookies contains fewer nutrients than dark or blackstrap molasses, most diners prefer its sweeter and milder flavor. It can also be used as a topping for pancakes or hot cereal.*

YIELD: 36 cookies                    SERVING SIZE: 1 cookie

| | WEIGHT | MEASURE |
|---|---|---|
| Butter-flavored vegetable oil cooking spray | — | — |
| Firmly packed light brown sugar | 4 oz | ½ c |
| Fat-free sour cream | 4 oz | ½ c |
| Light molasses | | ¼ c |
| Large egg | 2 oz | 1 |
| All-purpose flour | 6 oz | 1⅓ c |
| Ground cinnamon | | 1 tsp |
| Baking soda | | ½ tsp |
| Ground cloves | | ⅛ tsp |
| Ground nutmeg | | ⅛ tsp |
| Salt | | pinch |
| Firmly packed raisins | 3 oz | ½ c |

Preheat oven to 375 degrees F. Coat 2 or 3 baking sheets with cooking spray.

Combine brown sugar, sour cream, molasses, and egg in a medium bowl. Mix until well blended. For easy cleanup, measure the molasses in a cup that has been lightly coated with cooking spray.

Combine flour, cinnamon, baking soda, cloves, nutmeg, and salt in a medium bowl. Mix until well blended. Mix in raisins. Mix dry ingredients into liquid ingredients until blended.

Drop dough by teaspoonfuls onto prepared baking sheets. Bake until almost no indentation remains when touched, or about 8 minutes. Top with Lemon Powdered Sugar Frosting with Finely Grated Zest (page 221), if desired, and serve. Store between sheets of parchment or wax paper.

---

### NUTRITIONAL FACTS

Calories: 49 (4% from fat)
Fat: .2 g (.1 g sat, .1 g mono, 0 g poly)
Protein: .9 g and 89%

Carbohydrate: 10.9 g and 8%
Fiber: .3 g
Cholesterol: 5.9 mg
Iron: .5 mg

Sodium: 28.5 mg
Calcium: 16.7 mg
Diabetic Exchanges: ½ Other Carbohydrate

# Sugar Coated Molasses Jumbles

*Like fresh-baked gingerbread men, these ginger-spiced molasses cookies have an aroma that is reminiscent of the Christmas holidays and good times with family and friends. But these sugar-coated treats can be enjoyed without the guilt of their higher-fat counterparts.*

YIELD: 48 cookies                                 SERVING SIZE: 1 cookie

|                                              | WEIGHT | MEASURE         |
| -------------------------------------------- | ------ | --------------- |
| Butter-flavored vegetable oil cooking spray  | —      | —               |
| Granulated sugar, divided                    | 9 oz   | 1¼ c            |
| Light molasses                               |        | 1 c             |
| Prune purée (page 5) or prune baby food      | 4 oz   | ½ c             |
| All-purpose flour                            | 1 lb   | 3½ c (1¾ pt)    |
| Baking soda                                  |        | 2 tsp           |
| Salt                                         |        | 1 tsp           |
| Ground cinnamon                              |        | 1 tsp           |
| Ground ginger                                |        | ½ tsp           |
| Ground nutmeg                                |        | ¼ tsp           |
| Ground cloves                                |        | ¼ tsp           |

Preheat oven to 325 degrees F. Coat 2 or 3 baking sheets with cooking spray.

Combine 8 ounces (1 cup + 2 tablespoons) sugar, molasses, and prune purée in a large bowl. Mix until well blended. For easy cleanup, measure the molasses in a cup that has been lightly coated with cooking spray.

Combine flour, baking soda, salt, cinnamon, ginger, nutmeg, and cloves in a medium bowl. Mix until well blended.

Mix dry ingredients into molasses mixture until just blended. If dough is too dry, mix in decaffeinated coffee or water as needed, 1 teaspoon at a time.

Shape heaping teaspoonfuls of dough into balls. Roll in remaining 1 ounce (2 tablespoons) sugar. Place on prepared baking sheets about 2 inches apart. Flatten dough balls with a fork in crisscross pattern until ½ inch thick. Bake until set and bottoms are lightly browned, or about 10 minutes. Remove immediately to a wire rack to cool.

---

### NUTRITIONAL FACTS

Calories: 76 (1% from fat)  
Fat: .1 g  
Protein: 1 g and 5%  
Carbohydrate: 18 g and 93%  

Fiber: .4 g  
Cholesterol: 0 mg  
Iron: .8 mg  
Sodium: 81.5 mg  

Calcium: 16.8 mg  
Diabetic Exchanges: ½ Starch; ½ Other Carbohydrate

---

# Wholesome Apple Spice Oat Bars

*This recipe calls for quick-cooking rolled oats. They are equally as nutritious as long-cooking ("old fashioned") rolled oats. Long-cooking oats are oat groats that have been steamed and flattened with huge rollers. To reduce cooking time, quick-cooking rolled oats are made from groats that have been cut into several pieces before being steamed and rolled into thinner flakes. Don't replace quick-cooking oats with instant oats in this or other recipes; instant oats have been precooked and dried before being rolled.*

YIELD: 8-inch square bars  
SERVING SIZE: 2⅔-inch square  

SERVINGS: 9

| | WEIGHT | MEASURE |
|---|---|---|
| Butter-flavored vegetable oil cooking spray | — | — |
| Granulated sugar | 4 oz | ½ c |
| Large egg whites | 2½ oz | 2 |
| Prune purée (page 5) or prune baby food | 2 oz | ¼ c |
| All-purpose flour | 4 oz | ¾ c + 2 tbsp |
| Quick-cooking rolled oats | 1 oz | ¼ c |
| Baking powder | | ¾ tsp |
| Baking soda | | ¼ tsp |
| Salt | | ¼ tsp |
| Ground cinnamon | | ¼ tsp |
| Ground nutmeg | | ¼ tsp |
| Ground cloves | | ⅛ tsp |
| Peeled and cored apples diced into ¼-inch cubes | 4 oz | 1 c |

Preheat oven to 350 degrees F. Coat an 8-inch square baking pan with cooking spray.

Combine sugar, egg whites, and prune purée in a medium bowl. Mix until well blended.

Combine flour, oats, baking powder, baking soda, salt, cinnamon, nutmeg, and cloves in a small bowl. Mix until blended. Mix dry ingredients into liquid ingredients. Mix in apples until blended.

Spread evenly in prepared pan. Bake until a wooden pick inserted in center comes out clean, or 20 to 25 minutes. Cool bars in pan on a wire rack. Top with Orange Powdered Sugar Frosting with Finely Grated Zest (page 224), if desired. Cut into 9 squares and serve.

---

### NUTRITIONAL FACTS

| | | |
|---|---|---|
| Calories: 125 (3% from fat) | Carbohydrate: 28 g and 89% | Sodium: 153.4 mg |
| Fat: .4 g (.1 g sat, .1 g mono, .1 g poly) | Fiber: 1.1 g | Calcium: 29.6 mg |
| Protein: 2.7 g and 8% | Cholesterol: 0 mg | Diabetic Exchanges: 1 Starch; 1 Other Carbo- |
| | Iron: .8 mg | hydrate |

# Muffins, Biscuits, Pancakes, Coffee Cakes, and Other Breakfast Desserts

Applesauce Cinnamon White Whole Wheat Bread

Apricot Soy Bread Flavored with Orange

Baked Blueberry and Whole Wheat English Muffin
French Toast

Baked Oatmeal and Apple Breakfast Dessert

Blueberry Muffins Loaded with Blueberries

Blueberry Oat Bran Muffins Laced with Cinnamon

Bran Muffins Dotted with Raisins

Cornmeal Cranberry Drop Biscuits with Cinnamon

Cranberry Oat Muffins with a Hint of Orange

Cranberry White Whole Wheat Bread Flavored with Orange

Five-Spice Sugar-Free Cornmeal Muffins

Homestyle Banana Walnut Bread

Mincemeat Muffins Sprinkled with Walnuts

Pumpkin Bread Flavored with Aromatic Spices

Raspberry-Filled Crumble Coffee Cake

Whole Wheat Cinnamon Raisin Drop Biscuits

Whole Wheat Gingerbread Pancakes

Whole Wheat Oat Muffins Speckled with Dried Cherries

Whole Wheat Strawberry Pancakes Studded
with Strawberry Bits

# Applesauce Cinnamon White Whole Wheat Bread

*To enhance the nutritional profile of this quick bread, it is prepared with white whole wheat flour and enriched with applesauce and walnut bits toasted without fat. To toast nuts, cook in a dry nonstick skillet over medium heat, stirring constantly, until they just begin to become fragrant, or about 4 minutes. White whole wheat flour is whole grain flour with the fiber and extra nutrients of whole wheat flour but a milder taste. Egg whites replace the whole eggs. Usually, quick breads call for 4 to 8 tablespoons or more of margarine or butter per loaf. Here, the added fat of choice is a single tablespoon of monounsaturated olive oil.*

YIELD: 8½-inch loaf                                    SERVINGS: 16
SERVING SIZE: 1 slice (one-sixteenth loaf)

| | WEIGHT | MEASURE |
|---|---|---|
| Butter-flavored vegetable oil cooking spray | — | — |
| White whole wheat flour | 6 oz | 1¼ c |
| All-purpose flour | 3½ oz | ¾ c |
| Granulated sugar | 7 oz | 1 c |
| Baking powder | | 2 tsp |
| Ground cinnamon | | ½ tsp |
| Baking soda | | ½ tsp |
| Salt | | ¼ tsp |
| Chopped walnuts, toasted without fat | 2 oz | ½ c |
| Unsweetened applesauce | 8 oz | 1 c |
| Large egg whites | 2½ oz | 2 |
| Olive oil | | 1 tbsp |

Preheat oven to 350 degrees F. Coat an 8½-by-4½-by-2½-inch loaf pan with cooking spray.

Combine flours, sugar, baking powder, cinnamon, baking soda, and salt in a medium bowl. Mix until blended. Mix in nuts.

Combine applesauce, egg whites, and oil in a small bowl. Whisk until blended. Mix liquid ingredients into dry ingredients until just moist.

Spread batter evenly in prepared pan. Bake until a wooden pick inserted in center comes out clean, or about 50 minutes. Cool in pan for 10 minutes. Remove from pan to a wire rack to cool completely. Cut into 16 slices and serve.

---

### NUTRITIONAL FACTS

| | | |
|---|---|---|
| Calories: 145 (19% from fat) | Carbhydrate: 27.3 g and 72% | Sodium: 112.4 mg |
| Fat: 3.1 g (.3 g sat, 1.1 g mono, 1.4 g poly) | Fiber: 1.9 g | Calcium: 4.7 mg |
| Protein: 3.3 g and 9% | Cholesterol: 0 mg | Diabetic Exchanges: 1 Starch; ½ Other Carbo- |
| | Iron: .9 mg | hydrate; ½ Fruit; ½ Fat |

# Apricot Soy Bread Flavored with Orange

*The health benefits of eating soyfoods have been widely publicized. To create this sweet and tender quick bread dotted with apricot bits, part of the wheat flour was replaced with soy flour. Not only does soy flour add a sweet, pleasantly musty flavor to this bread, it improves its shelf life.*

YIELD: 8½-inch loaf                                           SERVINGS: 16
SERVING SIZE: 1 slice (one-sixteenth loaf)

| | WEIGHT | MEASURE |
|---|---|---|
| Butter-flavored vegetable oil cooking spray | — | — |
| Granulated sugar | 7 oz | 1 c |
| All-purpose flour | 4½ oz | 1 c |
| Soy flour | 3½ oz | 1 c |
| Dried apricot bits | 4 oz | ¾ c (15 apricot halves) |
| Baking powder | | 2 tsp |
| Baking soda | | ¼ tsp |
| Salt | | ¼ tsp |
| Large egg whites | 2½ oz | 2 |
| Fresh orange juice | | ¾ c |
| Finely grated orange zest | | 1 tbsp |
| Olive oil | | 1 tbsp |

Preheat oven to 350 degrees F. Coat an 8½-by-4½-by-2½-inch loaf pan with cooking spray.

Combine sugar, flours, apricots, baking powder, baking soda, and salt in a medium bowl. Mix until blended.

Combine egg whites, orange juice and zest, and oil in a small bowl. Whisk until blended. Mix liquid ingredients into dry ingredients until just moist.

Spread batter evenly in prepared pan. Bake until a wooden pick inserted in center comes out clean, or about 1 hour and 10 minutes. Cool in pan for 10 minutes. Remove from pan to a wire rack to cool completely. Cut into 16 slices and serve.

---

### NUTRITIONAL FACTS

| | | |
|---|---|---|
| Calories: 142 (14% from fat) | Carbohydrate: 27.2 g and 75% | Sodium: 92.8 mg |
| Fat: 2.2 g (.3 g sat, .6 g mono, .1 g poly) | Fiber: 1.8 g | Calcium: 18.1 mg |
| | Cholesterol: 0 mg | Diabetic Exchanges: ½ Starch; 1 Other Carbohydrate; ½ Fruit; ½ Fat |
| Protein: 3.9 g and 11% | Iron: 1.4 mg | |

---

# Baked Blueberry and Whole Wheat English Muffin French Toast

*Most people find it easy to eat the six to eleven daily servings of grain-based foods recommended in the USDA Food Guide Pyramid. The problem is making at least three of those whole grain foods. This whole wheat French toast recipe makes this simple, especially so because it can be prepared the day before. Another plus for this French toast recipe: Everyone, including the cook, gets to eat at the same time!*

YIELD: 8-inch square breakfast dessert   SERVINGS: 9
SERVING SIZE: 2⅔-inch square

| | WEIGHT | MEASURE |
|---|---|---|
| Butter-flavored vegetable oil cooking spray | — | — |
| Whole wheat English muffins, cut into 1-inch cubes | 12 oz | 6 whole |
| Block-style fat-free cream cheese, chilled and cut into 1-inch cubes | 8 oz | 1 c |
| Fresh or frozen unsweetened blueberries | 5 oz | 1 c |
| Evaporated fat-free milk | | 1 c |
| Large egg whites | 6¼ oz | 5 |
| Large egg | 2 oz | 1 |
| Honey | 2 oz | 2½ tbsp |
| Vanilla extract | | 1 tsp |

Coat an 8-inch square baking pan with cooking spray. Arrange half the muffin cubes in pan. Sprinkle cream cheese cubes over muffins. Sprinkle blueberries over cream cheese. Arrange remaining muffin cubes over blueberries.

Combine evaporated milk, egg whites, egg, honey, and vanilla in a small bowl. Whisk until blended. Pour evenly over muffin cubes, pressing to moisten with liquid. Cover with foil and refrigerate overnight.

Preheat oven to 350 degrees F. Place foil-covered pan in oven and bake for 30 minutes. Remove foil and bake until puffed and golden brown, or another 30 minutes. Cool on a wire rack at least 10 minutes. Cut into 9 pieces. Place on warm plates. Top with warm blueberry or pure maple syrup, honey, or fruit topping of choice, if desired, and serve.

---

### NUTRITIONAL FACTS

Calories: 168 (9% from fat)
Fat: 1.8 g (.6 g sat, .5 g mono, .4 g poly)
Protein: 11.9 g and 27%

Carbohydrate: 27.4 g and 63%
Fiber: 3 g
Cholesterol: 26.7 mg
Iron: 1.2 mg
Sodium: 449.5 mg

Calcium: 234.3 mg
Diabetic Exchanges: 1 Starch; ½ Other Carbohydrate; ½ Fruit; 1 Very Lean Meat

# Baked Oatmeal and Apple Breakfast Dessert

*Oats are one of the world's most nutritious grains. They are an excellent source of complex carbohydrates and provide more protein than bulgur wheat or brown rice. Furthermore, this whole grain supplies a substantial amount of iron and manganese along with good quantities of copper, folacin, vitamin E, and zinc. Here the oats are combined with diced apples and raisins, sweetened and flavored with fruit juice concentrate and a sprinkle of cinnamon, and enriched with creamy evaporated fat-free milk. The outcome is a wholesome sugar-free baked breakfast dessert.*

YIELD: 8-inch square dessert                    SERVINGS: 6
SERVING SIZE: 4-by-2⅔-inch piece

|  | WEIGHT | MEASURE |
|---|---|---|
| Butter-flavored vegetable oil cooking spray | — | — |
| Long-cooking ("old-fashioned") rolled oats | 3 oz | 1 c |
| Baking powder |  | 1 tsp |
| Ground cinnamon |  | ½ tsp |
| Thawed apple juice concentrate, undiluted |  | ¾ c |
| Evaporated fat-free milk |  | ½ c |
| Large egg whites | 2½ oz | 2 |
| Peeled and cored diced apples | 4 oz | 1 c |
| Firmly packed raisins | 2 oz | ⅓ c |

Preheat oven to 400 degrees F. Coat an 8-inch square baking pan with cooking spray.

Combine oats, baking powder, and cinnamon in a medium bowl. Mix until blended.

Combine apple juice concentrate, evaporated milk, and egg whites in a small bowl. Mix until blended. Mix liquid ingredients into dry ingredients until well blended.

Spread evenly in prepared pan. Bake for 20 minutes. Mix in apples and raisins. Continue baking until top is lightly browned, or about another 20 minutes. Cut into 6 pieces and serve. Top with fat-free plain yogurt or fat-free milk, if desired, and serve.

## NUTRITIONAL FACTS

| | | |
|---|---|---|
| Calories: 164 (7% from fat) | Carbohydrate: 34.3 g and 80% | Sodium: 90.7 mg |
| Fat: 1.3 g (.3 g sat, 0 g mono, .1 g poly) | Fiber: 2.6 g | Calcium: 76.1 mg |
| Protein: 5.4 g and 13% | Cholesterol: .9 mg | Diabetic Exchanges: ½ Starch; 1½ Fruits; ½ Skim Milk |
| | Iron: 1.2 mg | |

# Blueberry Muffins Loaded with Blueberries

*It may seem unusual for lemon zest to be an ingredient in blueberry muffins. Its purpose is not to give them a lemon flavor. Rather, it is to bring out the flavor of these golden brown-topped muffins dotted with plump and juicy dark blue berries.*

YIELD: 14 muffins                    SERVING SIZE: 1 muffin

| | WEIGHT | MEASURE |
|---|---|---|
| Butter-flavored vegetable oil cooking spray | — | — |
| Fat-free milk | | 1 c |
| Prune purée (page 5) or prune baby food | 6 oz | ¾ c |
| Granulated sugar | 5 oz | ¾ c |
| Large egg white | 1¼ oz | 1 |
| Olive oil | | 1 tbsp |
| All-purpose flour | 8 oz | 1¾ c |
| Baking powder | | 1 tbsp |
| Salt | | ½ tsp |
| Fresh or frozen unsweetened blueberries | 5 oz | 1 c |
| Finely grated lemon zest | | ½ tsp |

Preheat oven to 375 degrees F. Coat 14 muffin cups with cooking spray. Do not use paper liners as muffins will stick.

Combine milk, prune purée, sugar, egg white, and oil in a medium bowl. Whisk until well blended.

Combine flour, baking powder, and salt in a medium bowl. Mix until blended. Mix in blueberries and lemon zest. Mix liquid ingredients into dry ingredients until just moist.

Spoon batter into prepared muffin cups, dividing evenly. Bake until a wooden pick inserted in center comes out clean, or about 25 minutes. Remove muffins from pans immediately to a wire rack to cool. Serve warm or at room temperature.

---

### NUTRITIONAL FACTS

Calories: 152 (7% from fat)

Fat: 1.2 g (.2 g sat, .8 g mono, .2 g poly)

Protein: 2.9 g and 8%

Carbohydrate: 32.9 g and 85%

Fiber: 1.1 g

Cholesterol: .4 mg

Iron: 1.1 mg

Sodium: 149.6 mg

Calcium: 28.6 mg

Diabetic Exchanges: 1 Starch; ½ Other Carbohydrate; ½ Fruit

---

# Blueberry Oat Bran Muffins Laced with Cinnamon

*Oat bran is just as effective at reducing cholesterol levels as two widely prescribed cholesterol-lowering drugs and costs much less, according to a University of Maryland study cited in the University of California at Berkeley* Wellness Encyclopedia of Food and Nutrition. *These low-fat and cholesterol-free blueberry oat bran muffins offer a "sweet" alternative to drugs.*

YIELD: 14 muffins                                    SERVING SIZE: 1 muffin

|  | WEIGHT | MEASURE |
|---|---|---|
| Butter-flavored vegetable oil cooking spray | — | — |
| Oat bran | 6 oz | 1 c + 2 tbsp |
| All-purpose flour | 4 oz | ¾ c + 2 tbsp |
| Baking powder |  | 2 tsp |
| Ground cinnamon |  | 1 tsp |
| Salt |  | ¼ tsp |
| Fresh or frozen unsweetened blueberries | 5 oz | 1 c |
| Fat-free milk |  | 1 c |
| Granulated sugar | 6 oz | ¾ c + 2 tbsp |
| Prune purée (page 5) or prune baby food | 6 oz | ¾ c |
| Large egg white | 1¼ oz | 1 |

Preheat oven to 375 degrees F. Coat 14 muffin cups with cooking spray. Do not use paper liners as muffins will stick.

Combine oat bran, flour, baking powder, cinnamon, and salt in a large bowl. Mix until blended. Mix in blueberries.

Combine milk, sugar, prune purée, and egg white in a medium bowl. Whisk until well blended. Mix liquid ingredients into dry ingredients until just moist.

Spoon batter into prepared muffin cups, dividing evenly. Bake until a wooden pick inserted in center comes out clean, or 20 to 25 minutes. Remove muffins from pans to a wire rack immediately to cool. Serve warm or at room temperature.

---

### NUTRITIONAL FACTS

Calories: 132 (6% from fat)

Fat: 1.1 g (.2 g sat, .3 g mono, .4 g poly)

Protein: 4 g and 11%

Carbohydrate: 31.7 g and 83%

Fiber: 2.8 g

Cholesterol: .3 mg

Iron: 1.2 mg

Sodium: 125.8 mg

Calcium: 74 mg

Diabetic Exchanges: 1 Starch; ½ Other Carbohydrate; ½ Fruit

---

# Bran Muffins Dotted with Raisins

*If you like raisin bran cereal, these muffins are sure to become a favorite. Grab a carton of fat-free milk or yogurt, a piece of your favorite fruit, and one of these muffins for a quick-and-easy, low-fat breakfast on the go.*

YIELD: 14 muffins                                          SERVING SIZE: 1 muffin

| | WEIGHT | MEASURE |
|---|---|---|
| Butter-flavored vegetable oil cooking spray | — | — |
| Bran flakes | 3 oz | 2 c (1 pt) |
| Fat-free milk | | 1¼ c |
| Firmly packed light brown sugar | 4 oz | ½ c |
| Prune purée (page 5) or prune baby food | 3 oz | ¼ c + 2 tbsp |
| Large egg | 2 oz | 1 |
| Large egg white | 1¼ oz | 1 |
| All-purpose flour | 5 oz | 1 c + 2 tbsp |
| Baking powder | | 2 tsp |
| Ground cinnamon | | ¾ tsp |
| Salt | | ¼ tsp |
| Ground nutmeg | | ¼ tsp |
| Firmly packed raisins | 4 oz | ⅔ c |

Preheat oven to 375 degrees F. Coat 14 muffin cups with cooking spray. Do not use paper liners as muffins will stick.

Combine bran flakes and milk in a medium bowl. Stir well. Set aside.

Combine brown sugar, prune purée, egg, and egg white in a small bowl. Whisk until well blended.

Combine flour, baking powder, cinnamon, salt, and nutmeg in a large bowl. Mix until blended. Mix in raisins. Mix bran flake mixture and prune mixture into dry ingredients until just moist.

Spoon batter into prepared muffin cups, dividing evenly. Bake until a wooden pick inserted in center comes out clean, or about 25 minutes. Remove muffins from pans immediately to a wire rack to cool. Serve warm or at room temperature.

## NUTRITIONAL FACTS

| | | |
|---|---|---|
| Calories: 138 (5% from fat) | Carbohydrate: 30.3 g and 85% | Sodium: 154.9 mg |
| Fat: .8 g (.2 g sat, .3 g mono, .2 g poly) | Fiber: 1.5 g | Calcium: 45.4 mg |
| Protein: 3.6 g and 10% | Cholesterol: 15.6 mg | Diabetic Exchanges: 1 Starch; ½ Other Carbo- |
| | Iron: 2.7 mg | hydrate; ½ Fruit |

# Cornmeal Cranberry Drop Biscuits with Cinnamon

*The* Tufts University Health & Nutrition Letter *reported that the average American doesn't eat even one whole grain item a day. One way to increase whole grain consumption is to replace refined steel-ground cornmeal in recipes with stone-ground (water-ground) cornmeal. Stone-ground cornmeal, available in health-food stores and some supermarkets, is more nutritious because it retains some of the hull and germ of the corn. If you are unable to find it, substitute 6 ounces (1 cup) steel-ground, degermed yellow cornmeal in this recipe.*

YIELD: 16 biscuits                    SERVING SIZE: 1 biscuit

| | WEIGHT | MEASURE |
|---|---|---|
| Butter-flavored vegetable oil cooking spray | — | — |
| Stone-ground yellow cornmeal | 4½ oz | 1 c |
| All-purpose flour | 5½ oz | 1¼ c |
| Firmly packed light brown sugar | 2 oz | ¼ c |
| Baking powder | | 1 tbsp |
| Ground cinnamon | | 1 tsp |
| Baking soda | | ¼ tsp |
| Salt | | ¼ tsp |
| Stick margarine, chilled | 1½ oz | 3 tbsp |
| Sweetened dried cranberries | 4 oz | ¾ c |
| Unsweetened applesauce | 8 oz | 1 c |
| Large egg whites | 2½ oz | 2 |

Preheat oven to 425 degrees F. Coat a baking sheet with cooking spray.

Combine cornmeal, flour, brown sugar, baking powder, cinnamon, baking soda, and salt in a medium bowl. Mix until blended. Cut margarine into dry ingredients with a pastry blender or two knives until mixture resembles coarse crumbs. Mix in cranberries.

Combine applesauce and egg whites in a small bowl. Mix until blended. Mix liquid ingredients into dry ingredients until just moist soft dough forms.

Drop 16 biscuits by teaspoonfuls onto prepared baking sheets. Bake until golden brown, or about 15 minutes. For best results, serve immediately.

| NUTRITIONAL FACTS | | |
|---|---|---|
| Calories: 124 (18% from fat) | Carbohydrate: 23.3 g and 75% | Sodium: 136 mg |
| Fat: 2.5 g (.5 g sat, 1 g mono, .9 g poly) | Fiber: 1.6 g | Calcium: 8.1 mg |
| Protein: 2.1 g and 7% | Cholesterol: 0 mg | Diabetic Exchanges: 1 |
| | Iron: .8 mg | Starch; ½ Fruit; ½ Fat |

🌿

# Cranberry Oat Muffins with a Hint of Orange

*Like a steaming bowl of hot oatmeal topped with a sprinkle of sugar, a warm, sweet oat muffin dotted with dried cranberries is sure to hit the spot on a cold winter morning. This recipe calls for long-cooking ("old-fashioned") rolled oats. They work best, but if not available, quick oats can be substituted. Instant oats, however, make a poor substitute. Because instant oats are made from cut oat groats that have been softened in the precooking process, they don't provide enough substance and texture.*

YIELD: 14 muffins                    SERVING SIZE: 1 muffin

| | WEIGHT | MEASURE |
|---|---|---|
| Butter-flavored vegetable oil cooking spray | — | — |
| Long-cooking ("old-fashioned") rolled oats | 2 oz | ⅔ c |
| Fat-free milk | | 1 c |
| All-purpose flour | 5 oz | 1 c + 2 tbsp |
| Baking powder | | 1 tbsp |
| Salt | | ½ tsp |
| Sweetened dried cranberries | 4 oz | ¾ c |
| Finely grated orange zest | | 1 tsp |
| Granulated sugar | 3 oz | ¼ c + 2 tbsp |
| Large egg white | 1¼ oz | 1 |
| Prune purée (page 5) or prune baby food | 1 oz | 2 tbsp |
| Olive oil | | 1 tbsp |

Preheat oven to 375 degrees F. Coat 14 muffin cups with cooking spray. Do not use paper liners as muffins will stick.

Combine oats and milk in a small bowl. Stir well. Set aside.

Combine flour, baking powder, and salt in a medium bowl. Mix until blended. Mix in cranberries and orange zest.

Combine sugar, egg white, prune purée, and oil in a small bowl. Whisk until well blended. Mix prune mixture and soaked oats into dry ingredients until just moist.

Spoon batter into prepared muffin cups, dividing evenly. Bake until a wooden pick inserted in center comes out clean, or about 20 minutes. Remove muffins from pans immediately to a wire rack to cool. Serve warm or at room temperature.

---

### NUTRITIONAL FACTS

Calories: 124 (10% from fat)

Fat: 1.5 g (.3 g sat, .8 g mono, .1 g poly)

Protein: 2.6 g and 9%

Carbohydrate: 25.2 g and 82%

Fiber: 1.5 g

Cholesterol: .4 mg

Iron: .8 mg

Sodium: 146.6 mg

Calcium: 25.6 mg

Diabetic Exchanges: 1 Starch; ½ Other Carbohydrate; ½ Fat

# Cranberry White Whole Wheat Bread Flavored with Orange

*Researchers have called the shiny, tart red cranberries used in this bread the "jewels of good nutrition." Environmental Nutrition reported that in addition to fiber and vitamin C, cranberries are rich in antioxidants. Another nutritional benefit of this bread is that it is prepared with white whole wheat flour. Like whole wheat flour, it contains the bran and the germ along with the rest of the grain berry.*

YIELD: 8½-inch loaf

SERVINGS: 16

SERVING SIZE: 1 slice (one-sixteenth loaf)

| | WEIGHT | MEASURE |
|---|---|---|
| Butter-flavored vegetable oil cooking spray | — | — |
| Fresh or frozen unsweetened cranberries, ground | 5 oz | 1½ c |
| Granulated sugar, divided | 7 oz | 1 c |
| White whole wheat flour | 10 oz | 2 c (1 pt) |
| Baking powder | | 1 tbsp |
| Finely grated orange zest | | 1 tbsp |
| Salt | | ¼ tsp |
| Fat-free milk | | ¾ c |
| Large egg whites | 2½ oz | 2 |
| Olive oil | | 1 tbsp |

Preheat oven to 350 degrees F. Coat an 8½-by-4½-by-2½-inch loaf pan with cooking spray.

Combine cranberries and 2 ounces (¼ cup) sugar in a small bowl. Mix until blended.

Combine remaining 5 ounces (¾ cup) sugar, flour, baking powder, orange zest, and salt in a medium bowl. Mix until blended. Mix in cranberries until blended.

Combine milk, egg whites, and oil in a small bowl. Whisk until blended. Mix liquid ingredients into dry ingredients until just moist.

Spread batter evenly in prepared pan. Bake until a wooden pick inserted in center comes out clean, or about 1 hour. Cool in pan for 10 minutes. Remove from pan to a wire rack to cool completely. Cut into 16 slices and serve.

# Five-Spice Sugar-Free Cornmeal Muffins

*For an East-meets-West spin on cornmeal muffins, this fruit juice–sweetened, low saturated–fat, cholesterol-free version of the all-American favorite is seasoned with Chinese five-spice powder. This golden-brown spice mixture, available in most supermarkets and Asian markets, consists of five or six ground spices: cinnamon, cloves, fennel seed, star anise, and Szechwan peppercorns (or ginger or cardamom).*

YIELD: 12 muffins                    SERVING SIZE: 1 muffin

|  | WEIGHT | MEASURE |
|---|---|---|
| Butter-flavored vegetable oil cooking spray | — | — |
| Yellow cornmeal, degermed | 8 oz | 1¼ c |
| All-purpose flour | 4 oz | ¾ c + 2 tbsp |
| Baking powder |  | 2 tsp |
| Five-spice powder |  | 1 tsp |
| Baking soda |  | ½ tsp |
| Salt |  | ¼ tsp |
| Thawed apple juice concentrate, undiluted |  | 1 c |
| Large egg whites | 3¾ oz | 3 |
| Olive oil |  | 2 tbsp |

Preheat oven to 425 degrees F. Coat 12 muffin cups with cooking spray. Do not use paper liners as muffins will stick.

Combine cornmeal, flour, baking powder, five-spice powder, baking soda, and salt in a medium bowl.

Combine juice concentrate, egg whites, and oil in a small bowl. Whisk until well blended. Mix liquid ingredients into dry ingredients until just moist.

Spoon batter into prepared muffin cups, dividing evenly. Bake until a wooden pick inserted in center comes out clean, or about 12 minutes. Remove muffins from pan immediately to a wire rack to cool. Serve warm or at room temperature.

| NUTRITIONAL FACTS | | |
|---|---|---|
| Calories: 160 (18% from fat) | Carbohydrate: 29.8 g and 74% | Sodium: 164.6 mg |
| Fat: 3.2 g (.5 g sat, 2 g mono, .6 g poly) | Fiber: 1.7 g | Calcium: 8.7 mg |
| Protein: 3.5 g and 9% | Cholesterol: 0 mg | Diabetic Exchanges: 1½ Starches; ½ Fruit; ½ Fat |
| | Iron: 1.4 mg | |

# Homestyle Banana Walnut Bread

*Growing up, I looked forward to the bananas becoming overripe in our house. This usually meant that my mom would be serving her tender, moist, and oh-so-delicious banana bread for dinner. To speed up the ripening process, bake bright yellow-skinned bananas in their peels, in a 350-degree F oven, turning once, until black and the fruit is sweet, soft, and sticky, or about 15 minutes.*

YIELD: 8½-inch loaf                    SERVINGS: 16
SERVING SIZE: 1 slice (one-sixteenth loaf)

| | WEIGHT | MEASURE |
|---|---|---|
| Butter-flavored vegetable oil cooking spray | — | — |
| Chopped walnuts | 2 oz | ½ c |
| Puréed very ripe banana (4 medium-small) | 14 oz purée | 1¾ c |
| Granulated sugar | 6 oz | ¾ c + 2 tbsp |
| Large egg | 2 oz | 1 |
| Large egg white | 1¼ oz | 1 |
| Finely grated lemon zest | | ¾ tsp |
| All-purpose flour | 7 oz | 1½ c |
| Baking soda | | 1 tsp |
| Baking powder | | ¼ tsp |
| Salt | | ¼ tsp |

Preheat oven to 350 degrees F. Coat an 8½-by-4½-by-2½-inch loaf pan with cooking spray.

Toast nuts by cooking in a dry nonstick skillet over medium heat, stirring constantly until they just begin to become fragrant, or about 4 minutes.

Combine banana, sugar, egg, egg white, and lemon zest in a medium bowl. Whisk until well blended.

Combine flour, baking soda, baking powder, and salt in a medium bowl. Mix until blended. Mix in nuts. Mix liquid ingredients into dry ingredients until just moist.

Spread batter evenly in prepared pan. Bake until a wooden pick inserted in center comes out clean, or about 1 hour and 10 minutes. If top of loaf is becoming too brown, cover loosely with foil and continue baking. Cool in pan for 10 minutes. Remove from pan to a wire rack to cool completely. Cut into 16 slices and serve.

---

### NUTRITIONAL FACTS

Calories: 139 (18% from fat)

Fat: 2.9 g (.4 g sat, .5 g mono, 1.8 g poly)

Protein: 2.8 g and 8%

Carbohydrate: 26.5 g and 74%

Fiber: 1.2 g

Cholesterol: 15.4 mg

Iron: .8 mg

Sodium: 127.2 mg

Calcium: 9.2 mg

Diabetic Exchanges: ½ Starch; 1 Other Carbohydrate; ½ Fruit; ½ Fat

# Mincemeat Muffins Sprinkled with Walnuts

*Mincemeat is a rich and spicy fruit preserve. Old-fashioned versions typically contained both minced lean beef and beef suet. Today, most mincemeat is made without meat but to be sure, check the ingredient lists of commercially prepared products.*

YIELD: 12 muffins                    SERVING SIZE: 1 muffin

|  | WEIGHT | MEASURE |
|---|---|---|
| Butter-flavored vegetable oil cooking spray | — | — |
| Chopped walnuts | 2 oz | ½ c |
| Mincemeat | 10 oz | 1¼ c |
| Granulated sugar | 4 oz | ½ c |
| Fat-free milk |  | ¼ c |
| Fat-free plain yogurt | 2 oz | ¼ c |
| Large egg | 2 oz | 1 |
| Large egg white | 1¼ oz | 1 |
| Olive oil |  | 1 tbsp |
| All-purpose flour | 9 oz | 2 c (1 pt) |
| Baking powder |  | 1 tbsp |
| Finely grated orange zest |  | 1 tsp |
| Salt |  | ½ tsp |

Preheat oven to 375 degrees F. Coat 12 muffin cups with cooking spray. Do not use paper liners as muffins will stick.

Toast nuts by cooking in a dry nonstick skillet over medium heat, stirring constantly until they just begin to become fragrant, or about 4 minutes.

Combine mincemeat, sugar, milk, yogurt, egg, egg white, and oil in a medium bowl. Whisk until well blended.

Combine flour, baking powder, orange zest, and salt in a medium bowl. Mix until blended. Mix in nuts. Mix liquid ingredients into dry ingredients until just moist.

Spoon batter into prepared muffin cups, dividing evenly. Bake until a wooden pick inserted in center comes out clean, or about 20 minutes. Remove muffins from pan immediately to a wire rack to cool. Serve warm or at room temperature.

### NUTRITIONAL FACTS

Calories: 202 (21% from fat)

Fat: 4.9 g (.8 g sat, 1.7 g mono, 1.9 g poly)

Protein: 4.5 g and 9%

Carbohydrate: 37.4 g and 71%

Fiber: 1.8 g

Cholesterol: 17.9 mg

Iron: 2.3 mg

Sodium: 222.5 mg

Calcium: 31.8 mg

Diabetic Exchanges: ½ Starch; 1 Other Carbohydrate; ½ Fruit; ½ Low-Fat Milk; ½ Fat

# Pumpkin Bread Flavored with Aromatic Spices

*Until 1929, pumpkin was served only seasonally, as an autumn harvest and winter holiday specialty. That year canned solid-pack pumpkin was introduced, making it possible for us to enjoy our favorite pumpkin dishes such as this aromatic, low-fat quick bread year round. If cinnamon, allspice, nutmeg, and cloves are not among the spices in your collection, they can be replaced with 2 teaspoons of pumpkin pie spice in this recipe.*

YIELD: 8½-inch loaf     SERVINGS: 16
SERVING SIZE: 1 slice (one-sixteenth loaf)

| | WEIGHT | MEASURE |
|---|---|---|
| Butter-flavored vegetable oil cooking spray | — | — |
| Canned pumpkin | 10 oz | 1 c + 2 tbsp |
| Unpacked light brown sugar | 10 oz | 2 c (1 pt) |
| Large egg | 2 oz | 1 |
| Large egg white | 1¼ oz | 1 |
| Olive oil | | 1 tbsp |
| All-purpose flour | 8 oz | 1¾ c |
| Baking soda | | 1 tsp |
| Ground cinnamon | | 1 tsp |
| Ground allspice | | ¾ tsp |
| Salt | | ½ tsp |
| Ground nutmeg | | ½ tsp |
| Baking powder | | ¼ tsp |
| Ground cloves | | ⅛ tsp |

Preheat oven to 350 degrees F. Coat an 8½-by-4½-by-2½-inch loaf pan with cooking spray.

Combine pumpkin, brown sugar, egg, egg white, and oil in a medium bowl. Whisk until well blended.

Combine flour, baking soda, cinnamon, allspice, salt, nutmeg, baking powder, and cloves in a medium bowl. Mix until blended. Mix liquid ingredients into dry ingredients until just moist.

Spread batter evenly in prepared pan. Bake until a wooden pick inserted in center comes out clean, or about 1 hour and 5 minutes. If top of bread is becoming too brown after 45 minutes, cover loosely with foil and continue baking. Cool in pan for 10 minutes. Remove from pan to a wire rack to cool completely. Cut into 16 slices and serve.

---

### NUTRITIONAL FACTS

| | | |
|---|---|---|
| Calories: 139 (9% from fat) | Carbohydrate: 29.8 g and 84% | Sodium: 170.5 mg |
| Fat: 1.4 g (.3 g sat, .8 g mono, .2 g poly) | Fiber: 1 g | Calcium: 26.1 mg |
| Protein: 2.3 g and 6% | Cholesterol: 13.3 mg | Diabetic Exchanges: 1 Starch; 1 Other Carbohydrate |
| | Iron: 1.4 mg | |

---

# Raspberry-Filled Crumble Coffee Cake

*What makes this coffee cake special is its gooey raspberry filling and crumbly sugar topping. With frozen raspberries readily available year-round, there's no need to limit this breakfast treat to those few summer months when raspberries are in season.*

YIELD: 9-inch round cake                                    SERVINGS: 9
SERVING SIZE: 1 wedge (one-ninth 9-inch round)

## *FILLING*

| | WEIGHT | MEASURE |
| --- | --- | --- |
| Granulated sugar | 3 oz | scant ½ c |
| Cornstarch | ½ oz | 1⅔ tbsp |
| Fresh or frozen unsweetened raspberries | 5 oz | 1 c |
| Water | | ¼ c + 1 tbsp |
| Lemon juice | | 1 tsp |

## *COFFEE CAKE*

| | WEIGHT | MEASURE |
| --- | --- | --- |
| Butter-flavored vegetable oil cooking spray | — | — |
| Granulated sugar | 6 oz | ¾ c + 2 tbsp |
| Low-fat buttermilk | | ¾ c |
| Prune purée (page 5) or prune baby food | 3 oz | ¼ c + 2 tbsp |
| Large egg whites | 2½ oz | 2 |
| Vanilla extract | | ½ tsp |
| All-purpose flour | 6 oz | 1⅓ c |
| Baking powder | | 1 tsp |
| Baking soda | | ½ tsp |
| Salt | | ½ tsp |
| Ground cinnamon | | ½ tsp |
| Ground mace | | ⅛ tsp |

## *TOPPING*

| | WEIGHT | MEASURE |
| --- | --- | --- |
| Granulated sugar | 2 oz | ¼ c |
| All-purpose flour | 1½ oz | ⅓ c |
| Stick margarine, chilled | 1 oz | 2 tbsp |

For the filling: Combine sugar and cornstarch in a small bowl. Mix until blended. Combine raspberries and water in a small saucepan. Heat to boiling, then reduce heat. Stir in cornstarch mixture. Continue cooking and stirring until thickened and smooth. Remove from heat to cool. Mix in lemon juice.

For the cake: Preheat oven to 350 degrees F. Coat a 9-inch round cake pan with cooking spray.

Combine sugar, buttermilk, prune purée, egg whites, and vanilla in a medium bowl. Mix until well blended.

Combine flour, baking powder, baking soda, salt, cinnamon, and mace in a medium bowl. Mix until blended. Mix liquid ingredients into dry ingredients just until moist. Spread half the batter in prepared pan. Spread cooled filling over batter. Spoon small mounds of remaining batter over filling and spread out as much as possible with a spatula.

For the topping: Combine sugar and flour in a small bowl. Mix until blended. Cut in margarine with a pastry blender or two knives until mixture resembles coarse crumbs. Sprinkle topping evenly over batter. Bake until a wooden pick inserted in center comes out clean, or about 40 minutes. Cool in pan on a wire rack. Cut into 9 wedges and serve.

---

### NUTRITIONAL FACTS

| | | |
|---|---|---|
| Calories: 293 (9% from fat) | Carbohydrate: 63 g and 85% | Calcium: 36.2 mg |
| Fat: 3.1 g (.7 g sat, 1.2 g mono, 1 g poly) | Fiber: 2.1 g | Diabetic Exchanges: 1½ Starches; 2 Other |
| Protein: 4.3 g and 6% | Cholesterol: 1.3 mg | Carbohydrates; ½ Fruit; ½ Fat |
| | Iron: 1.5 mg | |
| | Sodium: 292 mg | |

---

# Whole Wheat Cinnamon Raisin Drop Biscuits

*Because these lightly sweetened, golden-brown, crisp-crusted tender biscuits require no kneading or rolling, they are easy to make. Fragrant with cinnamon and hinting of banana, they are heavenly warm out of the oven drizzled with powdered sugar frosting.*

YIELD: 20 biscuits                    SERVING SIZE: 1 biscuit

|  | WEIGHT | MEASURE |
|---|---|---|
| Butter-flavored vegetable oil cooking spray | — | — |
| Whole wheat pastry flour or whole wheat flour | 4 oz | scant 1 c |
| All-purpose flour | 4 oz | ¾ c + 2 tbsp |
| Firmly packed light brown sugar | 4 oz | ½ c |
| Baking powder |  | 1 tbsp |
| Ground cinnamon |  | 1 tbsp |
| Baking soda |  | ¼ tsp |
| Salt |  | ¼ tsp |
| Stick margarine, chilled | 1½ oz | 3 tbsp |
| Firmly packed raisins | 4 oz | ⅔ c |
| Puréed very ripe banana (2 medium-large) | 8 oz purée | 1 c |
| Large egg whites | 2 | 2½ oz |
| Unsifted powdered sugar | 2 oz | ½ c |
| Fat-free milk |  | 2 tsp or as needed |

Preheat oven to 400 degrees F. Coat 2 baking sheets with cooking spray.

Combine flours, brown sugar, baking powder, cinnamon, baking soda, and salt in a medium bowl. Mix until blended. Cut margarine into dry ingredients with a pastry blender or two knives until mixture resembles coarse crumbs. Mix in raisins.

Combine banana and egg whites in a small bowl. Mix until well blended. Mix liquid ingredients into dry ingredients until just moist soft dough forms.

Drop 20 biscuits by teaspoonfuls onto prepared baking sheets. Bake until golden brown, or about 12 minutes.

Combine powdered sugar and milk in a small bowl. Beat until smooth and of frosting consistency. Frost biscuits warm out of the oven and serve immediately.

---

### NUTRITIONAL FACTS

Calories: 118 (14% from fat)

Fat: 2 g (.4 g sat, .8 g mono, .6 g poly)

Protein: 2.1 g and 7%

Carbohydrate: 24.3 g and 79%

Fiber: 1.5 g

Cholesterol: 0 mg

Iron: .9 mg

Sodium: 108.7 mg

Calcium: 16.7 mg

Diabetic Exchanges: ½ Starch; ½ Other Carbohydrate; ½ Fruit; ½ Fat

# Whole Wheat Gingerbread Pancakes

*With all the taste of gingerbread, these aromatic whole wheat pancakes make a nutritious breakfast or brunch alternative to deep-fried donuts or butter-laden sweet rolls.*

YIELD: fifteen 4-inch pancakes  
SERVING SIZE: three 4-inch pancakes  

SERVINGS: 5

| | WEIGHT | MEASURE |
|---|---|---|
| Whole wheat pastry flour or whole wheat flour | 6 oz | 1⅓ c |
| Baking powder | | 2½ tsp |
| Ground cinnamon | | ¾ tsp |
| Ground ginger | | ½ tsp |
| Ground nutmeg | | ¼ tsp |
| Salt | | ¼ tsp |
| Ground cloves | | ⅛ tsp |
| Fat-free milk | | 1½ c |
| Unsweetened applesauce | 2 oz | ¼ c |
| Light molasses | | ¼ c |
| Large egg whites | 2½ oz | 2 |
| Butter-flavored vegetable oil cooking spray | — | — |

Combine flour, baking powder, cinnamon, ginger, nutmeg, salt, and cloves in a medium bowl. Mix until blended.

Combine milk, applesauce, molasses, and egg whites in a small bowl. For easy cleanup, measure the molasses in a cup that has been lightly coated with cooking spray. Whisk until blended. Pour wet ingredients over dry ingredients. Gently whisk just until blended. For thinner pancakes, mix in additional milk. For thicker pancakes, mix in additional flour. (Note: The additional milk or flour will not be included in the nutrition analysis.)

Coat a large nonstick griddle or skillet with cooking spray. Place over medium heat until hot. Pour from a pitcher or spoon 3-tablespoon portions of batter onto the hot griddle or skillet. Cook until bubbles appear on surface of pancakes and bottoms are golden brown, or about 2 minutes. Turn and cook until other sides are golden brown, or about 2 minutes. Repeat, using all batter.

Serve immediately on warm plates or keep warm in 200 degree F oven while you finish cooking the rest. Spoon fruit topping over or drizzle with warm pure maple syrup, if desired.

| NUTRITIONAL FACTS | | |
| --- | --- | --- |
| Calories: 208 (3% from fat) | Carbohydrate: 43.1 g and 80% | Calcium: 163.2 mg |
| Fat: .7 g (.2 g sat, .1 g mono, .3 g poly) | Fiber: 4.5 g | Diabetic Exchanges: 1½ Starches; ½ Other |
| Protein: 9.1 g and 17% | Cholesterol: 1.6 mg | Carbohydrate; ½ Fruit; |
| | Iron: 2.7 mg | ½ Skim Milk |
| | Sodium: 306.3 mg | |

# Whole Wheat Oat Muffins Speckled with Dried Cherries

*These muffins contain lots of goodies, but it is the dried cherries that make them ideal for Presidents' Day. They can be transformed into Fourth of July specialties by preparing with dried blueberries or featured on Thanksgiving studded with dried apricot bits. At Christmas, mix in dried cranberries and for every day, date bits or raisins are familiar favorites. These muffins are also excellent without any dried fruit.*

YIELD: 17 muffins                    SERVING SIZE: 1 muffin

| | WEIGHT | MEASURE |
|---|---|---|
| Long-cooking ("old-fashioned") rolled oats | 4 oz | 1⅓ c |
| Low-fat buttermilk | | 2 c (1 pt) |
| Butter-flavored vegetable oil cooking spray | — | — |
| Firmly packed light brown sugar | 6 oz | ¾ c |
| Large egg whites | 2½ oz | 2 |
| Prune purée (page 5) or prune baby food | 1 oz | 2 tbsp |
| Whole wheat pastry flour or whole wheat flour | 7 oz | 1⅔ c |
| Baking powder | | 2 tsp |
| Baking soda | | 1 tsp |
| Salt | | 1 tsp |
| Sweetened dried cherries | 4 oz | ¾ c |

Combine oats and buttermilk in a medium bowl. Stir well. Cover and refrigerate for 6 hours or overnight.

Preheat oven to 375 degrees F. Coat 17 muffin cups with cooking spray. Do not use paper liners as muffins will stick.

Combine brown sugar, egg whites, and prune purée in a large mixing bowl. Beat until well blended.

Combine flour, baking powder, baking soda, and salt in a small bowl. Mix until blended. Mix in dried cherries. Mix dry ingredients and soaked oats into liquid ingredients until just moist.

Spoon batter into prepared muffin cups, dividing evenly. Bake until a wooden pick inserted in center comes out clean, or about 20 minutes. Remove muffins to a wire rack to cool or serve warm.

---

### NUTRITIONAL FACTS

Calories: 141 (6% from fat)

Fat: 1 g (.3 g sat, .2 g mono, .2 g poly)

Protein: 4.4 g and 12%

Carbohydrate: 29.8 g and 82%

Fiber: 2.6 g

Cholesterol: 1.8 mg

Iron: 1.1 mg

Sodium: 281 mg

Calcium: 51.6 mg

Diabetic Exchanges: 1½ Starches; ½ Other Carbohydrate

# Whole Wheat Strawberry Pancakes Studded with Strawberry Bits

*For a breakfast that is "berry" hard to beat, mix up a batch of these light golden brown pancakes. They are laced with bits of America's favorite berries, strawberries, swirled with strawberry spread, and splashed with almond extract.*

YIELD: twelve 4-inch pancakes                    SERVINGS: 4
SERVING SIZE: three 4-inch pancakes

| | WEIGHT | MEASURE |
|---|---|---|
| Whole wheat pastry flour or whole wheat flour | 2 oz | ½ c |
| All-purpose flour | 2 oz | ¼ c + 3 tbsp |
| Baking powder | | 2 tsp |
| Salt | | ¼ tsp |
| Hulled and diced fresh ripe strawberries | 5 oz | 1 c |
| Fat-free milk | | ½ c |
| 100%-fruit strawberry spread | 3 oz | ¼ c |
| Almond extract | | ½ tsp |
| Large egg whites | 2½ oz | 2 |
| Cream of tartar | | pinch |
| Butter-flavored vegetable oil cooking spray | — | — |

Combine flours, baking powder, and salt in a medium bowl. Mix until blended. Mix in strawberries.

Combine milk, strawberry spread, and almond extract in a small bowl. Mix until well blended. Pour wet ingredients over dry ingredients. Gently whisk just until blended.

Beat egg whites with an electric mixer until foamy. Add cream of tartar. Continue beating until stiff but not dry. Gently fold egg whites into batter. For thinner pancakes, mix in additional milk. For thicker pancakes, mix in additional all-purpose flour. (Note: The additional milk or flour will not be included in the nutrition analysis.)

Coat a large nonstick griddle or skillet with cooking spray. Place over medium heat until hot. Pour from a pitcher or spoon 3-tablespoon portions of batter onto the hot griddle or skillet. Cook until bubbles appear on surface of pancakes and bottoms are golden brown, or about 2 minutes. Turn and cook until other sides are golden brown, or about 2 minutes. Repeat, using all batter.

Serve immediately on warm plates or keep warm in 200 degree F oven while you finish cooking the rest. Drizzle warm pure maple syrup over or top with a dollop of vanilla reduced-fat ice cream, if desired.

| NUTRITIONAL FACTS | | |
|---|---|---|
| Calories: 168 (2% from fat) | Carbohydrate: 35.1 g and 82% | Sodium: 306.7 mg |
| Fat: .5 g (.1 g sat, .1 g mono, .2 g poly) | Alcohol: .2 g and 1% | Calcium: 52.2 mg |
| Protein: 6.5 g and 15% | Fiber: 3 g | Diabetic Exchanges: 1 Starch; ½ Other Carbohydrate; ½ Fruit; ½ Skim Milk |
| | Cholesterol: .6 mg | |
| | Iron: 1.5 mg | |

# Pies, Tarts, and Cheesecakes

Apple Pie Just Like Grandma's

Banana Lovers' Firm Custard Pie

Blackberry Snow Tart in Graham Cracker Crumb Crust

Homestyle Pumpkin Pie with Tofu

Honey-Glazed Fresh Fruit Melange in Phyllo Tart Shells

Honey-Sweetened Sweet Potato Pie with a Splash
of Bourbon Whiskey

Hot Peach Tart on Oat Bran Crust

Lemon-Flavored Cheesecake in Graham Cracker Crumb Crust

Lemon Meringue Pie in Whole Wheat Crust

Lime Chiffon Angel Pie in Graham Cracker Crumb Crust

Mango Cream Cheese Pie Decorated with Sliced Mangoes

Oatmeal Raisin Pie with Pure Maple Syrup

Peach Pie Topped with Lemon Marshmallow Meringue

Pineapple Custard Cream Meringue Pie

Pumpkin Chiffon Pie Dashed with Orange
in Corn Flake Crumb Crust

Red Cherry Pie Splashed with Amaretto

Rhubarb Strawberry Pie with a Hint of Orange and Cinnamon

Sweet Potato Cheesecake Drizzled with Apple-Flavored
Caramel Glaze

Tropical Fruit Curd Decorated with Strawberries
in Meringue Pastry Shell

# Apple Pie Just Like Grandma's

*One thing I remember about my grandma: She baked the best apple pie around. Everybody who tasted Grandma's pie would rave about it. This apple pie is a lower-fat and lower-calorie version of Grandma's. It begins with a reduced-fat whole wheat crust. Next, thinly sliced Granny Smith apples are coated in a mixture of granulated and brown sugars, corn syrup, and just the right amount of cinnamon and nutmeg. The apples are spooned into the crust and sprinkled with a corn flake crumb topping.*

YIELD: 9-inch pie                                        SERVINGS: 8
SERVING SIZE: 1 wedge (one-eighth pie)

### CRUST

| | WEIGHT | MEASURE |
|---|---|---|
| Whole Wheat Pastry Crust (page 177), unbaked | | 1 recipe |

### TOPPING

| | WEIGHT | MEASURE |
|---|---|---|
| Corn flake crumbs | 3 oz | ¾ c |
| Firmly packed light brown sugar | 3 oz | ¼ c + 2 tbsp |
| Thawed apple juice concentrate, undiluted | | 2½ tbsp |
| Stick margarine, melted | ½ oz | 1 tbsp |

### FILLING

| | WEIGHT | MEASURE |
|---|---|---|
| Peeled and thinly sliced Granny Smith or other tart apples | 1¾ lb | 5½ c (1⅜ qt) |
| Granulated sugar | 3 oz | scant ½ c |
| Firmly packed light brown sugar | 2 oz | ¼ c |
| All-purpose flour | 1 oz | 3 tbsp |
| White corn syrup | 1 oz | 1½ tbsp |
| Ground cinnamon | | 1 tsp |
| Ground nutmeg | | ⅛ tsp |

For the crust: Prepare and set aside. Preheat oven to 375 degrees F.

For the topping: Combine corn flake crumbs and brown sugar in a small bowl. Drizzle juice concentrate and melted margarine over crumb mixture. Mix until crumbs are evenly moistened. Set aside.

For the filling: Combine apples, sugars, flour, corn syrup, cinnamon, and nutmeg in a large bowl. Toss gently until well mixed. Spoon apple slices into the unbaked pastry crust. Sprinkle corn flake topping over.

Bake until apples are tender and crust and topping are golden brown, or about 50 minutes. If topping is becoming too brown, cover loosely with foil. Cool until pie juices have thickened, or about 1 hour. Cut into 8 wedges and serve. Top with a scoop of vanilla low-fat ice cream, if desired.

---

NUTRITIONAL FACTS

Calories: 365 (19% from fat)
Fat: 7.8 g (1.5 g sat, 3.2 g mono, 2.4 g poly)
Protein: 3.5 g and 4%

Carbohydrate: 72 g and 77%
Fiber: 3.6 g
Cholesterol: 0 mg
Iron: 3.9 mg
Sodium: 294.2 mg

Calcium: 36.7 mg
Diabetic Exchanges: 1½ Starches; 1½ Other Carbohydrates; 1½ Fruits; 1½ Fats

---

# Banana Lovers' Firm Custard Pie

*Americans eat more bananas than any other fruit: about 28 pounds each year. Nutritionally, bananas have a lot going for them. At about 95 calories for an average-size banana, they are very low in sodium and fat, have more potassium (by weight) than practically any other fruit, are richer in carbohydrates (by weight) than most fruits, and contain quite high amounts of several vitamins and additional minerals. When dessert calls for more than just a simple banana, offer this rich reduced-fat banana custard pie. A firm vanilla custard is layered with thick, sweet banana slices and baked in a crunchy graham cracker crumb crust.*

YIELD: 9-inch pie                                    SERVINGS: 8
SERVING SIZE: 1 wedge (one-eighth pie)

| | WEIGHT | MEASURE |
|---|---|---|
| Graham Cracker Crumb Crust and Topping (page 170) | | 1 recipe (9-inch crust + topping) |
| Fat-free sweetened condensed milk | | ¾ c + 2 tbsp |
| Fat-free sour cream | 10 oz | 1 c + 2 tbsp |
| Low-fat milk | | ¼ c |
| Ripe bananas, peeled | 1½ lb as purchased | 4 medium |

Prepare crust and topping and set aside. Preheat oven to 375 degrees F.

Combine condensed milk, sour cream, and milk in a small bowl. Beat until blended.

Cut bananas into ¼-inch-thick slices and place bananas in crust. Pour condensed milk mixture over bananas.

Bake until just set, or about 15 minutes. Cool. Sprinkle with graham cracker crumb topping. Refrigerate until serving time. Cut into 8 wedges and serve.

---

### NUTRITIONAL FACTS

Calories: 427 (22% from fat)

Fat: 10.7 g (1.8 g sat, 4.2 g mono, 3.3 g poly)

Protein: 8.3 g and 8%

Carbohydrate: 76.3 g and 70%

Fiber: .9 g

Cholesterol: 2.9 mg

Iron: 2 mg

Sodium: 336 mg

Calcium: 276.5 mg

Diabetic Exchanges: 2 Starches; 1½ Other Carbohydrates; 1½ Fruits; 2 Fats

---

# Blackberry Snow Tart in Graham Cracker Crumb Crust

*The American poet Walt Whitman wrote that blackberries "adorned heaven." To assure that this dessert is a "heaven on earth" experience, follow these tips when handling the blackberries for this pie: (1) Select plump, bright, and deep purplish blackberries. Avoid blackberries with*

*their hulls still attached. They have been picked before they are mature and will be tart in flavor. (2) Discard any moldy blackberries, as they cannot be cleaned and will contaminate the rest. (3) Fresh blackberries are best if used immediately. If this is not possible, refrigerate the berries in a paper or plastic container with holes or open spaces for up to two days. Top wrappers should be pierced or very loosely fastened to allow air to circulate. (4) Wash blackberries only when you are ready to use them, as they deteriorate once wet. (5) Wash blackberries in a colander or strainer so that cold water runs through them. Place them on paper towels to dry.*

YIELD: 9-inch pie                                    SERVINGS: 8
SERVING SIZE: 1 wedge (one-eighth pie)

|  | WEIGHT | MEASURE |
|---|---|---|
| Graham Cracker Crumb Crust (page 170), or one 6-oz reduced-fat graham cracker crust |  | 1 recipe |
| Unflavored gelatin |  | 1 envelope (scant 1 tbsp) |
| Thawed white grape juice concentrate, undiluted |  | ¾ c |
| Fresh or frozen unsweetened blackberries | 8 oz | 1⅔ c |
| Fat-free plain yogurt | 4 oz | ½ c |
| Finely grated orange zest |  | ½ tsp |
| Large egg whites, at room temperature | 3¾ oz | 3 |
| Cream of tartar |  | ¼ tsp |
| Evaporated fat-free milk, chilled in freezer 30 minutes |  | ¼ c |

Prepare crust and set aside.

Sprinkle gelatin over juice concentrate in a small saucepan. Let stand until softened, or about 5 minutes. Cook over low heat, stirring to dissolve gelatin.

Purée blackberries in a blender or food processor until smooth. Strain through a fine mesh strainer; discard seeds. Combine purée, yogurt, orange zest, and dissolved gelatin mixture in a medium bowl. Mix until well blended. Cover surface with plastic wrap and chill until mixture mounds slightly.

Combine egg whites and cream of tartar in a medium mixing bowl. Beat with an electric mixer until stiff peaks form. Gently fold beaten egg whites into blackberry mixture.

Beat partially frozen evaporated milk with an electric mixer in a large mixing bowl until soft peaks form. Gently fold blackberry-egg white mixture into evaporated milk. Refrigerate filling until it mounds slightly. Mound in crust. Chill until set, or about 3 hours. Cut into 8 wedges. Garnish with additional blackberries and mint sprigs, if desired, and serve. Store refrigerated.

---

### NUTRITIONAL FACTS

Calories: 229 (26% from fat)

Fat: 6.7 g (1.2 g sat, 2.8 g mono, 2.3 g poly)

Protein: 5.2 g and 9%

Carbohydrate: 38.3 g and 65%

Fiber: 2.2 g

Cholesterol: .6 mg

Iron: 1.2 mg

Sodium: 222.6 mg

Calcium: 65.4 mg

Diabetic Exchanges: 1½ Starches; 1 Fruit; 1 Fat

---

# Homestyle Pumpkin Pie with Tofu

*The health benefits of soy foods have been well publicized. Soybeans are an excellent source of high-quality protein and are rich in calcium, iron, zinc, several of the B vitamins, and fiber. In addition, soybeans contain a wealth of phytochemicals. It appears that even a serving a day may be sufficient to produce health benefits. If soy foods are a new experience for your guests, let them try this pumpkin pie before telling them it is made with tofu. When you announce your secret ingredient, their surprise will be followed by compliments.*

YIELD: 9-inch pie

SERVING SIZE: 1 wedge (one-eighth pie)

SERVINGS: 8

| | WEIGHT | MEASURE |
|---|---|---|
| Whole Wheat Pastry Crust (page 177), unbaked | | 1 recipe |
| Low-fat extra-firm silken tofu | 12.3-oz package | |
| Canned pumpkin | 15-oz can | 1⅔ c |
| Unpacked light brown sugar | 5 oz | 1 c |
| Large egg whites, lightly beaten | 2½ oz | 2 |
| Ground cinnamon | | 1½ tsp |
| Ground ginger | | ¾ tsp |
| Ground cloves | | ⅛ tsp |

Prepare crust and set aside. Preheat oven to 425 degrees F.

Combine tofu and pumpkin in a food processor or blender. Blend until smooth. Place in a bowl. Add brown sugar, egg whites, cinnamon, ginger, and cloves. Whisk until well blended.

Pour into unbaked pastry crust. Bake for 15 minutes, then reduce oven heat to 350 degrees F. Bake until a knife inserted in center comes out clean, or about another 40 minutes. Cool completely. Cut into 8 wedges. Top with a small scoop of vanilla reduced-fat ice cream, if desired, and serve. Store refrigerated.

---

### NUTRITIONAL FACTS

Calories: 210 (26% from fat)
Fat: 6.4 g (1.3 g sat, 2.6 g mono, 2 g poly)
Protein: 6.5 g and 12%

Carbohydrate: 34.1 g and 62%
Fiber: 3.2 g
Cholesterol: 0 mg
Iron: 2.1 mg
Sodium: 213.1 mg

Calcium: 65.4 mg
Diabetic Exchanges: 1 Starch; 1 Other Carbohydrate; 1 Vegetable; 1 Fat

# Honey-Glazed Fresh Fruit Melange in Phyllo Tart Shells

*For those with a sweet tooth yet a concern for fat and calories, these single-serving-size pastries are a dream come true. Light, crisp phyllo shells are filled with bright red strawberries, fragrant golden peach slices, and juicy yellow pineapple cubes all glazed in a light honey syrup splashed with brandy and flavored with mint.*

YIELD: 4 tarts

SERVING SIZE: 1 tart

|  | WEIGHT | MEASURE |
|---|---|---|
| Light and Crisp Phyllo Tart Shells (page 172), baked |  | 1 recipe |
| Brandy |  | ¼ c |
| Honey |  | 3 tbsp |
| Minced mint leaves |  | 1 tbsp |
| Hulled and sliced fresh ripe strawberries | 5 oz | scant 1 c |
| ¼-inch-thick peeled ripe peach slices | 5 oz | scant 1 c |
| Fresh ripe pineapple cubes | 5 oz | scant 1 c |

Prepare tart shells and set aside.

Place brandy in a small saucepan. Cook over medium heat until reduced to 1 tablespoon. Add honey. Mix until blended. Stir in mint.

At serving time, combine fruit and brandy-honey mixture in a bowl. Mix gently until fruit is well coated. Spoon into tart shells and serve.

---

### NUTRITIONAL FACTS

Calories: 131 (10% from fat)
Fat: 1.5 g (.2 g sat, .2 g mono, .2 g poly)
Protein: 1 g and 3%

Carbohydrate: 28.8 g and 81%
Alcohol: 1.2 g and 6%
Fiber: 2.1 g
Cholesterol: 0 mg
Iron: .6 mg

Sodium: 24.4 mg
Calcium: 12.6 mg
Diabetic Exchanges: ½ Starch; ½ Other Carbohydrate; 1 Fruit

# Honey-Sweetened Sweet Potato Pie with a Splash of Bourbon Whiskey

*In the United States, dark-skinned and bright orange–fleshed sweet pota-toes are often erroneously called yams. Sometimes even canned and frozen sweet potatoes are labeled yams. While sweet potatoes and true yams can be similar in size and shape, the two vegetables are from different plant species, and true yams can range from small potato size to over 7½ feet in length and 120 pounds in weight. Thus, to be technically correct, this is a sweet potato, not a yam, pie.*

YIELD: 9-inch pie SERVINGS: 8
SERVING SIZE: 1 wedge (one-eighth pie)

| | WEIGHT | MEASURE |
| --- | --- | --- |
| Whole Wheat Pastry Crust (page 177), un-baked | | 1 recipe |
| Mashed peeled sweet potatoes, cooked with-out salt, or drained and mashed canned sweet potatoes | 18 oz | 2¼ c (1⅛ pt) |
| Evaporated fat-free milk | | 1 ½ c |
| Honey | 12 oz | 1 c |
| Large egg whites, lightly beaten | 3¾ oz | 3 |
| Bourbon whiskey | | 2 tbsp |
| Ground cinnamon | | 1½ tsp |
| Ground allspice | | ¼ tsp |
| Ground nutmeg | | ⅛ tsp |

Prepare crust and set aside. Preheat oven to 425 degrees F.

Combine sweet potatoes, evaporated milk, honey, egg whites, whiskey, cinnamon, allspice, and nutmeg in a blender or food processor. Blend un-til smooth and well mixed. Pour into pastry crust.

Bake for 15 minutes, then reduce oven heat to 350 degrees F. Bake un-til a knife inserted in center comes out clean, or about another 50 minutes. Cool completely. Cut into 8 wedges. Top with a small scoop of vanilla fat-free frozen yogurt, if desired, and serve. Store refrigerated.

---

### NUTRITIONAL FACTS

Calories: 343 (15% from fat)

Fat: 6.2 g (1.2 g sat, 2.6 g mono, 1.9 g poly)

Protein: 8.3 g and 9%

Carbohydrate: 67.2 g and 75%

Alcohol: .3 g and 1%

Fiber: 2.8 g

Cholesterol: 1.9 mg

Iron: 1.9 mg

Sodium: 272.3 mg

Calcium: 179.1 mg

Diabetic Exchanges: 1½ Starches; 2 Other Carbohydrates; ½ Fruit; ½ Skim Milk; 1 Fat

---

# Hot Peach Tart on Oat Bran Crust

*These individual tarts allow the artist in the baker to "come out and play." They call for thinly sliced golden peaches to be beautifully arranged on individual thin, flat oat bran rounds, baked until the peaches are tender and the pastry is golden brown and then drizzled with warm raspberry spread. While they are time consuming, they are not difficult to make. If successful, they look and taste stunning and are an ideal light and healthy dessert when peaches are in season.*

YIELD: 6 tarts　　　　　　　　　　SERVING SIZE: one 4½-inch tart

|  | WEIGHT | MEASURE |
|---|---|---|
| All-purpose flour | 3½ oz | ¾ c |
| Oat bran | 1 oz | ¼ c |
| Stick margarine, chilled | 2 oz | ¼ c |
| Very cold water |  | 2 tbsp |
| Fresh ripe peaches | 16 oz as purchased | 3 medium/2 large |
| Ground cinnamon |  | 1½ tsp |
| 100%-fruit raspberry spread |  | 3 tbsp |

Combine flour and oat bran in a small bowl. Mix until blended. Cut margarine into mixture with a pastry blender or two knives until mixture resembles coarse crumbs. Slowly add water, tossing with a fork until flour is moistened without being wet. If mixture seems dry or crumbly, sprinkle in another teaspoon cold water. The dough should not be damp or sticky.

Press mixture together with a fork. Turn dough out onto a piece of parchment or wax paper and press firmly together into a ball. Divide dough into 6 equal pieces. Gently shape each piece into a flattened round. Refrigerate 1 to 24 hours.

Preheat oven to 400 degrees F.

Roll each dough ball with a rolling pin between 2 sheets of parchment or wax paper into an ⅛-inch-thick round. Peel off top paper. Trim each round with a sharp knife or pastry wheel into a perfect circle, using a 4½-inch plate or a pattern as a guide.

Pick each dough circle up with parchment paper. Turn onto a baking sheet. Prick with a fork. Bake to partially cook, or about 5 minutes. Cool.

Peel the peaches: Blanch them in boiling water for 20 to 60 seconds and then place in ice water or under cold running water until completely cooled. The skins should slip off easily. Slice peaches thinly. Or use 12 ounces (2 cups) thinly sliced frozen unsweetened peaches, if desired.

Arrange peach slices pinwheel style on cooled pastry, covering almost to edge. Sprinkle with cinnamon. Return to oven until peaches are tender and pastry golden brown, or about 15 minutes.

When tarts are almost baked, melt raspberry spread in a small saucepan over low heat. Remove tarts from oven. Drizzle each with ½ tablespoon raspberry spread. Transfer with a spatula to 6 warm dessert plates and serve immediately.

| NUTRITIONAL FACTS | | |
|---|---|---|
| Calories: 166 (32% from fat) | Carbohydrate: 26.9 g and 61% | Sodium: 96.5 mg |
| Fat: 6.3 g (1.4 g sat, 2.6 g mono, 1.9 g poly) | Fiber: 2.6 g | Calcium: 17.1 mg |
| Protein: 3 g and 7% | Cholesterol: 0 mg | Diabetic Exchanges: 1 Starch; ½ Other Carbohydrate; ½ Fruit; 1 Fat |
| | Iron: 1.3 mg | |

# Lemon-Flavored Cheesecake in Graham Cracker Crumb Crust

*This light and healthy cheesecake is light on the palate, as well as low in cholesterol and saturated fat. A crumbly graham cracker crumb crust is topped with a moist and creamy lemon-flavored filling and finished with Summer-Fresh Three Berry Sauce. In comparison to average store brands, this cheesecake has 50 percent less fat.*

YIELD: 9-inch cheesecake      SERVINGS: 16
SERVING SIZE: 1 wedge (one-sixteenth cheesecake)

| | WEIGHT | MEASURE |
|---|---|---|
| Butter-flavored vegetable oil cooking spray | — | — |
| Stick margarine | 1½ oz | 3 tbsp |
| Graham cracker crumbs | 6 oz | 1½ c |
| Thawed apple juice concentrate, undiluted | | ¼ c + 2 tbsp |
| Block-style fat-free cream cheese, softened | 1 lb | 2 c (1 pt) |
| Fat-free sweetened condensed milk | 14-oz can | |
| Fat-free sour cream | 8 oz | 1 c |
| Large egg whites | 5 oz | 4 |
| Fresh lemon juice | | ¼ c + 2 tbsp |
| Granulated sugar | 1 oz | 2 tbsp |
| Finely grated lemon zest | | 1½ tbsp |
| Vanilla extract | | 1 tsp |
| Salt | | ⅛ tsp |
| Summer-Fresh Three Berry Sauce (page 228) | | 1 recipe |

Preheat oven to 325 degrees F. Coat a 9-inch springform pan with cooking spray.

Melt margarine in a small saucepan. Add cracker crumbs and juice concentrate. Mix until crumbs are evenly moistened. Press evenly into bottom and about 1½ inches up sides of prepared pan. Set aside.

Combine cream cheese, condensed milk, sour cream, egg whites, lemon juice, sugar, lemon zest, vanilla, and salt in a food processor or blender. Blend until smooth and creamy. Pour over cracker crumbs.

Bake until set, or about 50 minutes. Cool in pan on a wire rack. Remove sides of pan. Refrigerate until chilled, or several hours. Cut into 16 wedges. Drizzle with Summer-Fresh Three Berry Sauce. Garnish with lemon twists and mint sprigs, if desired, and serve. To make twisted fluted lemon slices, peel lemon from top to bottom in alternate strips with a channel knife (stripper) or small peeler. Slice fruit thin and cut each slice ¾ of the way across and twist open.

---

### NUTRITIONAL FACTS

Calories: 197 (15% from fat)
Fat: 3.3 g (.6 g sat, 1.4 g mono, 1.1 g poly)
Protein: 9.1 g and 19%

Carbohydrate: 32.1 g and 66%
Fiber: .4 g
Cholesterol: 3.8 mg
Iron: .5 mg
Sodium: 297.6 mg

Calcium: 179.6 mg
Diabetic Exchanges: 1 Starch; ½ Other Carbohydrate; ½ Fruit; ½ Skim Milk; ½ Fat

---

# Lemon Meringue Pie in Whole Wheat Crust

*As a child, I'd love it when my mother was in the mood for lemon meringue pie. She'd make a rich lemon filling, thickening and enriching it with lots of egg yolks and finishing it with butter. This lemon pie filling contains neither the butter nor the egg yolks called for in the traditional recipe. Nor does it require standing and cooking over the range as my mother's version did. Rather, this rich-tasting, smooth lemon-flavored filling is created by blending fat-free sweetened condensed milk with freshly squeezed lemon juice and finely grated lemon zest. Thickening occurs because the lemon reacts with the milk.*

YIELD: 9-inch pie                                               SERVINGS: 8
SERVING SIZE: 1 wedge (one-eighth pie)

| | WEIGHT | MEASURE |
|---|---|---|
| Whole Wheat Pastry Crust (page 177), baked | | 1 recipe |
| Fat-free sweetened condensed milk | 14-oz can | |
| Fresh lemon juice | | ¾ c |
| Finely grated lemon zest | | 1⅓ tbsp |
| Yellow food coloring | | few drops (optional) |
| Meringue Topping for Pie (page 175) | | 1 recipe |

Prepare pastry crust and set aside. Reduce oven heat to 350 degrees F.

Combine condensed milk, lemon juice and zest, and food coloring (if using) in a medium bowl. Mix until thickened. Pour mixture into pastry crust. Prepare meringue topping and spread meringue topping over filling. Seal to pastry crust. This helps prevent shrinkage.

Bake until lightly browned, or about 15 to 20 minutes. Cool completely. Cut into 8 wedges and serve. Store refrigerated.

---

### NUTRITIONAL FACTS

| | | |
|---|---|---|
| Calories: 265 (20% from fat) | Carbohydrate: 47.3 g and 69% | Sodium: 213 mg |
| Fat: 6.1 g (1.1 g sat, 2.5 g mono, 1.8 g poly) | Fiber: 1.6 g | Calcium: 154.4 mg |
| Protein: 7.3 g and 11% | Cholesterol: 3.3 mg | Diabetic Exchanges: 2 Starch; ½ Other Carbohydrate; ½ Fruit; 1 Fat |
| | Iron: .6 mg | |

---

# Lime Chiffon Angel Pie in Graham Cracker Crumb Crust

*A crunchy reduced-fat and -calorie graham cracker crumb crust is filled with a refreshing lime chiffon and served with a bright red raspberry sauce. In addition to sounding good, this pie is made with lots of good-for-you ingredients. They include calcium and protein-rich, fat-free yogurt; vitamin C–packed lime juice; and high-protein, fat-free, cholesterol-free egg whites. Additionally, the filling is sweetened with fruit juice concentrate rather than refined white sugar.*

YIELD: 9-inch pie                          SERVINGS: 8
SERVING SIZE: 1 wedge (one-eighth pie)

|  | WEIGHT | MEASURE |
|---|---|---|
| Graham Cracker Crumb Crust (page 170) or one 6-oz reduced-fat graham cracker crust | | 1 recipe |
| Unflavored gelatin | | 1 tbsp |
| Thawed white grape juice concentrate, undiluted | | 1¼ c |
| Fat-free plain yogurt | 6½ oz | ¾ c |
| Fresh lime juice | | ¼ c |
| Finely grated lime zest | | 1 tbsp |
| Large egg whites, at room temperature | 2½ oz | 2 |
| Cream of tartar | | ¼ tsp |
| Raspberry Sauce Sweetened with Fruit Juice (page 227) | | 1 recipe |

Prepare crust and set aside.

Sprinkle gelatin over juice concentrate in a medium saucepan. Let stand until softened, or about 5 minutes. Cook over low heat, stirring to dissolve gelatin.

Remove from heat. Mix in yogurt and lime juice and zest until well blended. Cover and chill until mixture mounds on a spoon.

Combine egg whites and cream of tartar in a small mixing bowl. Beat with an electric mixer until stiff peaks form. Gently fold egg whites into lime-yogurt mixture until completely blended.

Spread filling evenly in crust. Chill until set (don't touch the filling), or about 3 hours. While pie is chilling, prepare the raspberry sauce. Cut into 8 wedges. Drizzle each piece with 3 tablespoons Raspberry Sauce Sweetened with Fruit Juice and serve. Store refrigerated.

---

### NUTRITIONAL FACTS

| | | |
|---|---|---|
| Calories: 243 (24% from fat) | Carbohydrate: 43 g and 69% | Sodium: 212.3 mg |
| Fat: 6.6 g (1.2 g sat, 2.8 g mono, 2.2 g poly) | Fiber: .8 g | Calcium: 45.2 mg |
| Protein: 4.4 g and 7% | Cholesterol: .5 mg | Diabetic Exchanges: 1½ Starch; 1½ Fruits; 1 Fat |
| | Iron: 1.1 mg | |

# Mango Cream Cheese Pie
# Decorated with Sliced Mangoes

*For a Mexican touch to this pie, fragrant mangoes are blended with fat-free sour cream and fat-free cream cheese, then sweetened with brown sugar and spooned into a crunchy corn flake crumb crust. After making the pie's filling, there is no need to bake, simply refrigerate until chilled.*

*To prepare the mangoes, score the skin lengthwise in 4 to 6 places. Pull the skin off. Cut the flesh from each side of the large central pit and chop or slice.*

YIELD: 9-inch pie             SERVINGS: 8
SERVING SIZE: 1 wedge (one-eighth pie)

|  | WEIGHT | MEASURE |
| --- | --- | --- |
| Corn Flake Crumb Crust (page 168) | | 1 recipe |
| Unflavored gelatin | | 1 tbsp |
| Mango nectar | | 1 c |
| Fresh ripe, peeled mangoes, ½ chopped and ½ sliced | 2 lbs as purchased | 2 large/4 small |
| Fat-free sour cream | 2 oz | ¼ c |
| Block-style fat-free cream cheese | 6 oz | ¾ c |
| Firmly packed light brown sugar | 4 oz | ½ c |
| Lemon juice | | 2 tbsp |
| Vanilla extract | | ½ tsp |
| Almond extract | | ⅛ tsp |

Prepare crust and set aside.

Sprinkle gelatin over mango nectar in a small saucepan. Let stand until softened, or about 5 minutes. Cook over low heat, stirring to dissolve gelatin. Set aside.

Combine chopped mango and sour cream in a blender or food processor. Blend until smooth. Add cream cheese, brown sugar, lemon juice, vanilla, almond extract, and gelatin mixture. Blend until smooth.

Pour into crumb crust. Refrigerate until chilled, or 3 to 4 hours. Decorate with mango slices. Cut into 8 wedges. Garnish with mint sprigs, if desired, and serve.

NUTRITIONAL FACTS

| | | |
|---|---|---|
| Calories: 275 (11% from fat) | Carbohydrate: 58 g and 81% | Sodium: 285.5 mg |
| Fat: 3.5 g (.8 g sat, 1.5 g mono, 1 g poly) | Alcohol: .1 g and 0% | Calcium: 82.8 mg |
| Protein: 6 g and 8% | Fiber: 2.3 g | Diabetic Exchanges: ½ Starch; 1 Other Carbo- |
| | Cholesterol: 3 mg | hydrate; 2 Fruits; ½ |
| | Iron: 3.3 mg | Skim Milk; ½ Fat |

# Oatmeal Raisin Pie with Pure Maple Syrup

*There's no need to reserve oatmeal for breakfast. It's equally delicious in this pie. Best yet, oats are one of the most nutritious grains. These whole grains contain both soluble and insoluble fiber. It's the soluble fiber, called beta glucan, that experts believe is responsible for oats' cholesterol-lowering benefits. The* UC Berkeley Wellness Letter *also reported that there is evidence that fiber may help control blood sugar and improve insulin sensitivity, too, and thus benefit people with insulin resistance or diabetes.*

*Be sure to use pure maple syrup in this pie. As noted in* The Essential Cook Book *by Caroline Conran, Terence Conran, and Simon Hopkinson, "some syrups are made by God and others are made by man. Maple syrup is among the former."*

YIELD: 9-inch pie                    SERVINGS: 8
SERVING SIZE: 1 wedge (one-eighth pie)

| | WEIGHT | MEASURE |
|---|---|---|
| Graham Cracker Crumb Crust (page 170) or one 6-oz reduced-fat graham cracker crust | | 1 recipe |
| Pure maple syrup | 9 oz | ¾ c |
| Large egg whites | 3 | 3¾ oz |
| Quick-cooking oats | 7½ oz | 2¼ c (1⅛ pt) |
| Firmly packed raisins | 4 oz | ⅔ c |
| All-purpose flour | | 1 tbsp |
| Ground cinnamon | | 1 tsp |

Prepare crust and set aside. Preheat oven to 325 degrees F.

Combine maple syrup and egg whites in a medium bowl. Mix until well blended. Add oats, raisins, flour, and cinnamon. Mix until well blended.

Spoon into crust. Bake until the top is golden brown and filling just set in center, or about 45 minutes. Cool completely. Cut into 8 wedges. Top with a scoop of vanilla fat-free frozen yogurt, if desired, and serve.

---

### NUTRITIONAL FACTS

Calories: 371 (20% from fat)
Fat: 8.4 g (1.5 g sat, 3.3 g mono, 2.8 g poly)
Protein: 7.3 g and 8%

Carbohydrate: 68.2 g and 72%
Fiber: 3.4 g
Cholesterol: 0 mg
Iron: 2.5 mg
Sodium: 206.1 mg

Calcium: 48.9 mg
Diabetic Exchanges: 2½ Starches; 1 Other Carbohydrate; 1 Fruit; 1½ Fats

---

# Peach Pie Topped with Lemon Marshmallow Meringue

*To give peach pie a healthy new twist, a reduced-fat whole wheat crust is topped with beta carotene–rich peach slices, then coated in fruit juice glaze and topped with golden lemon marshmallow meringue. The citrus-*

*flavored airy egg-white topping makes a refreshing complement to the golden peach filling. When fresh peaches aren't readily available, frozen peaches work well in this pie, too.*

YIELD: 9-inch pie                                               SERVINGS: 8
SERVING SIZE: 1 wedge (one-eighth pie)

| | WEIGHT | MEASURE |
|---|---|---|
| Whole Wheat Pastry Crust (page 177), baked | | 1 recipe |
| Peeled and thinly sliced fresh ripe peaches | 1 lb 10 oz | 4½ c (1⅛ qt) |
| Thawed white grape juice concentrate, undiluted | | 1 c |
| Cornstarch | | ¼ c |
| Finely grated lemon zest | | 2 tsp |
| Lemon Marshmallow Meringue Topping (page 171) | | 1 recipe |

Prepare crust and set aside. Lower oven heat to 350 degrees F.

To peel the peaches, blanch them in boiling water for 20 to 60 seconds and then place them in ice water or under cold running water until completely cooled. The skins should slip off easily. Place peaches in a baking pan. Cover and bake until tender, or about 30 minutes. Remove from oven and reset to 450 degrees F.

Combine juice concentrate and cornstarch in a small saucepan. Mix until smooth. Cook over medium heat, stirring until thickened.

Add juice in peach pan to thickened juices. Mix until blended. Add thickened juices and lemon zest to peaches. Mix until peaches are evenly coated.

Spoon filling into baked pastry crust. Prepare Lemon Marshmallow Meringue Topping and spread over warm filling, sealing to crust. Bake until lightly browned, or 3 to 5 minutes. Set to cool until juices have thickened, or about 1 hour. Cut into 8 wedges and serve. Store refrigerated.

---

### NUTRITIONAL FACTS

| | | |
|---|---|---|
| Calories: 310 (17% from fat) | Carbohydrate: 62.4 g and 77% | Sodium: 182.1 mg |
| Fat: 6.2 g (1.2 g sat, 2.6 g mono, 1.9 g poly) | Fiber: 3.5 g | Calcium: 23.8 mg |
| Protein: 4.6 g and 6% | Cholesterol: 0 mg | Diabetic Exchanges: 1 Starch; 1 Other Carbohydrate; 2 Fruits; 1 Fat |
| | Iron: .8 mg | |

# Pineapple Custard Cream Meringue Pie

*From its golden brown fat- and cholesterol-free meringue topping to its sweet and creamy, fat- and cholesterol-free pineapple filling and reduced-fat whole wheat pastry crust, this pie meets all the criteria for a tasty and healthy dessert.*

YIELD: 9-inch pie                                                     SERVINGS: 8
SERVING SIZE: 1 wedge (one-eighth pie)

| | WEIGHT | MEASURE |
|---|---|---|
| Whole Wheat Pastry Crust (page 177), baked | | 1 recipe |
| Granulated sugar | 6 oz | ¾ c + 2 tbsp |
| All-purpose flour | | 2 tbsp |
| Salt | | ⅛ tsp |
| Fat-free sour cream | 8½ oz | 1 c |
| Large egg whites | 3 ¾ oz | 3 |
| Crushed pineapple canned in juice, drained, reserving ½ c juice | 20-oz can | |
| Meringue Topping for Pie (page 175) | | 1 recipe |

Prepare crust and set aside. Reduce oven heat to 350 degrees F.

Combine sugar, flour, and salt in a medium saucepan. Mix well. Stir in sour cream, egg whites, and ½ cup reserved pineapple juice. Mix until blended.

Simmer over medium-low heat, stirring, until thick. Remove from heat. Mix in pineapple. Transfer to a medium storage container. Cover surface with plastic wrap. Refrigerate until just cool. Spoon into pastry crust.

Prepare meringue topping and spread over filling, sealing to pastry crust. This helps prevent shrinkage. Bake until meringue is lightly browned, or about 15 minutes. Cool completely. Cut into 8 wedges and serve. Store refrigerated.

## NUTRITIONAL FACTS

Calories: 271 (19% from fat)

Fat: 6 g (1.1 g sat, 2.6 g mono, 1.8 g poly)

Protein: 6.4 g and 9%

Carbohydrate: 49.3 g and 71%

Fiber: 2 g

Cholesterol: 0 mg

Iron: .9 mg

Sodium: 240.7 mg

Calcium: 59.6 mg

Diabetic Exchanges: 2 Starches; ½ Other Carbohydrate; ½ Fruit; 1 Fat

# Pumpkin Chiffon Pie Dashed with Orange in Corn Flake Crumb Crust

*There's no need to wait until Thanksgiving to put pumpkin pie on the menu. This chilled, fluffy pumpkin chiffon pie with a hint of orange is the perfect light dessert for a hot summer day. Rather than the expected graham cracker crumb crust, this beta carotene–rich pie filling is complemented by a crunchy corn flake crumb crust.*

YIELD: 9-inch pie

SERVINGS: 8

SERVING SIZE: 1 wedge (one-eighth pie)

| | WEIGHT | MEASURE |
|---|---|---|
| Corn Flake Crumb Crust (page 168) | | 1 recipe |
| Evaporated fat-free milk | | ¼ c + 2 tbsp |
| Unflavored gelatin | | 1 envelope |
| | | (scant 1 tbsp) |
| Canned pumpkin | 18 oz | 2 c (1 pt) |
| Large egg whites, divided | 5 oz | 4 |
| Firmly packed light brown sugar | 4 oz | ½ c |
| Thawed orange juice concentrate, undiluted | | 1 tbsp |
| Finely grated orange zest | | 1 tsp |
| Ground cinnamon | | ¼ tsp |
| Ground ginger | | ⅛ tsp |
| Ground nutmeg | | ⅛ tsp |
| Cream of tartar | | ¼ tsp |
| Granulated sugar | 3 oz | scant ½ c |

Prepare crust, reserving 2 tablespoons corn flake crumbs to sprinkle over top of pie. Refrigerate until use.

Place evaporated milk in a small bowl. Sprinkle gelatin over. Let stand until softened, or about 5 minutes.

Combine pumpkin, 2½ ounces (2) egg whites, brown sugar, orange juice concentrate, orange zest, cinnamon, ginger, and nutmeg in a medium bowl. Whisk until well blended. Place in a saucepan of barely simmering water. Cook, stirring, until thick. Stir in soaked gelatin until dissolved. Cover and chill until mixture mounds on a spoon.

Combine remaining egg whites and cream of tartar in a medium mixing bowl. Beat with an electric mixer until soft peaks form. Slowly beat in granulated sugar. Continue beating until stiff glossy peaks form.

Gently fold whipped egg whites into pumpkin mixture. Spread filling evenly in crust. Sprinkle reserved 2 tablespoons corn flake crumbs over filling. Chill until set, or about 3 hours. Cut into 8 wedges and serve. Store refrigerated.

---

### NUTRITIONAL FACTS

Calories: 280 (9% from fat)
Fat: 2.9 g (.6 g sat, 1.3 g mono, .9 g poly)
Protein: 4.6 g and 6%

Carbohydrate: 60.4 g and 84%
Fiber: 1.4 g
Cholesterol: .4 mg
Iron: 3.6 mg

Sodium: 297.3 mg
Calcium: 71 mg
Diabetic Exchanges: 1 Starch; 2 Other Carbohydrates; 1 Fruit; ½ Fat

# Red Cherry Pie Splashed with Amaretto

*Fruit pie fillings are frequently thickened with flour or cornstarch. The result is a gluey texture, dull color, and lackluster flavor. For a crystal-clear and vibrant-tasting filling with a more delicate texture, this cherry pie is thickened with quick-cooking tapioca. If only pearl tapioca is available, make your own quick cooking tapioca by processing it in a blender or food processor until the granules are broken into small bits.*

YIELD: 9-inch pie             SERVINGS: 8
SERVING SIZE: 1 wedge (one-eighth pie)

| | WEIGHT | MEASURE |
|---|---|---|
| Reduced-Fat and Cholesterol-Free Pastry Crust (page 176) unbaked | | ½ recipe (9-inch crust + cutouts) |
| Tart pitted and drained red cherries, canned in water, divided | 1 lb 7 oz | 2 14½-oz cans, |
| Minute tapioca | 1 oz | 3 tbsp |
| Ground allspice | | ⅛ tsp |
| Ground cinnamon | | ⅛ tsp |
| Thawed white grape juice concentrate, undiluted | | 1⅔ c |
| Amaretto (almond-flavored liqueur) | | 3 tbsp |
| Red food coloring | | 12 drops (optional) |

Prepare crust and set aside. Preheat oven to 450 degrees F.

Combine two-thirds drained cherries with tapioca, allspice, and cinnamon in a medium bowl. Toss lightly to mix. Add grape juice concentrate, amaretto, and food coloring (if using). Mix well. Let stand about 15 minutes.

Spoon cherry mixture into pastry crust. Spoon remaining cherries over. Top with pastry cutouts.

Bake for 10 minutes, then reduce oven heat to 350 degrees F and bake until crust is golden brown, or about 40 minutes longer. If crust's edges are becoming too brown, cover with foil and continue baking. Set to cool until juices have thickened, or about 1 hour. Cut into 8 wedges and serve.

## NUTRITIONAL FACTS

| | | |
|---|---|---|
| Calories: 269 (20% from fat) | Carbohydrate: 51.1 g and 75% | Iron: 2.2 mg |
| Fat: 6.2 g (1.2 g sat, 2.6 g mono, 2 g poly) | Alcohol: .3 g and 1% | Sodium: 157.1 mg |
| Protein: 3 g and 4% | Fiber: 1.6 g | Calcium: 22.2 mg |
| | Cholesterol: 0 mg | Diabetic Exchanges: 1 Starch; 2½ Fruits; 1 Fat |

# Rhubarb Strawberry Pie with a Hint of Orange and Cinnamon

*I can't imagine growing up without a patch of rhubarb in the backyard. From the rose-colored stalks' first appearance in early spring through its midsummer growing season, my mother was busy turning the tart shoots into cinnamon-sugar encrusted homey rhubarb cake, rhubarb sauce splashed with orange, and pebbly topped aromatic rhubarb muffins. This recipe is dedicated to those wonderful childhood memories.*

YIELD: 9-inch pie        SERVINGS: 8
SERVING SIZE: 1 wedge (one-eighth pie)

|  | WEIGHT | MEASURE |
|---|---|---|
| Reduced-Fat and Cholesterol-Free Pastry Crust (page 176), unbaked |  | ½ recipe (9-inch crust + cutouts) |
| 1-inch pieces fresh or frozen unsweetened rhubarb | 1¼ lb | 5 c (1¼ qt) |
| Hulled and quartered fresh ripe strawberries | 13 oz | 2¼ c (1⅛ pt) |
| Granulated sugar | 10 oz | scant 1½ c |
| Cornstarch |  | ¼ c + 1 tbsp |
| Vanilla extract |  | 2 tsp |
| Ground cinnamon |  | 1 tsp |
| Finely grated orange zest |  | 1 tsp |
| Large egg white | ¾ oz | ½ (1½ tbsp) |
| Water |  | 1½ tsp |
| Granulated sugar |  | 1 tsp |

Prepare crust and set aside. Preheat oven to 400 degrees F.

Combine rhubarb, strawberries, sugar, cornstarch, vanilla, cinnamon, and orange zest in a large bowl. Mix gently.

Spoon into unbaked pastry crust. Top with pastry cutouts. To divide egg white in half, whip lightly and then divide. Beat half egg white and water together in a small bowl. Brush on pastry cutouts. Sprinkle lightly with 1 teaspoon sugar.

Bake until crust is golden brown, or 50 to 60 minutes. Set to cool until juices have thickened. Cut into 8 wedges and serve.

---

### NUTRITIONAL FACTS

Calories: 318 (17% from fat)
Fat: 6.2 g (1.2 g sat, 2.6 g mono, 2 g poly)
Protein: 3.2 g and 4%

Carbohydrate: 64 g and 79%
Fiber: 3.1 g
Cholesterol: 0 mg
Iron: 1.4 mg
Sodium: 155.2 mg

Calcium: 77.4 mg
Diabetic Exchanges: 1 Starch; 2½ Other Carbohydrates; 1 Fruit; 1 Fat

# Sweet Potato Cheesecake Drizzled with Apple-Flavored Caramel Glaze

*Sweet potatoes are one of the most nutritious vegetables. The orange-fleshed tubers are rich in beta-carotene; a good source of fiber, manganese, and copper; and contain only about 120 calories per 5-inch potato. Their creamy texture and sweet taste add richness to this fruit juice–sweetened cheesecake without fat or cholesterol.*

YIELD: 9-inch cheesecake

SERVINGS: 16

SERVING SIZE: 1 wedge (one-sixteenth cheesecake)

| | WEIGHT | MEASURE |
|---|---|---|
| Butter-flavored vegetable oil cooking spray | — | — |
| Stick margarine | 1½ oz | 3 tbsp |
| Graham cracker crumbs | 6 oz | 1½ c |
| Thawed apple juice concentrate, undiluted | | ¼ c + 2 tbsp |
| Puréed peeled sweet potatoes, cooked without salt, or drained and puréed canned sweet potatoes | 8 oz | 1 c |
| All-purpose flour | | 1 tbsp |
| Brandy | | 1 tbsp |
| Ground cinnamon | | ¼ tsp |
| Ground nutmeg | | ⅛ tsp |
| Ground allspice | | ⅛ tsp |
| Ground cloves | | pinch |
| Block-style fat-free cream cheese | 1 lb | 2 c |
| Unpacked light brown sugar | 7 oz | 1⅓ c |
| Large egg whites | 3¾ oz | 3 |

Preheat oven to 350 degrees F. Coat a 9-inch springform pan with cooking spray.

Melt margarine in a small saucepan. Add cracker crumbs and juice concentrate. Mix until crumbs are evenly moistened. Press evenly into bottom and about 1½ inches up sides of prepared pan. Set aside.

Combine sweet potato purée, flour, brandy, cinnamon, nutmeg, all-spice, and cloves in a medium bowl. Mix until well blended. Set aside.

Place cream cheese in a medium mixing bowl. Beat with an electric mixer until smooth and creamy. Gradually beat in brown sugar until smooth.

Add egg whites one at a time, mixing on low speed. Beat until just blended. Gradually add sweet potato mixture, beating until smooth. Pour into crumb-lined pan.

Bake until center appears set but jiggles slightly when gently shaken, or about 50 minutes. Leave cake in oven another 30 minutes with oven turned off and door open at least 4 inches. Cool cake in pan on a wire rack. Remove sides of pan. Refrigerate several hours or until chilled. Cut into 16 wedges. Spoon on Apple-Flavored Caramel Glaze with a Splash of Brandy (page 214), if desired, and serve.

---

### NUTRITIONAL FACTS

Calories: 164 (18% from fat)
Fat: 3.3 g (.6 g sat, 1.4 g mono, 1.1 g poly)
Protein: 6 g and 15%

Carbohydrate: 27.6 g and 67%
Fiber: .6 g
Cholesterol: 2.2 mg
Iron: .9 mg
Sodium: 250.8 mg

Calcium: 105.1 mg
Diabetic Exchanges: ½ Starch; 1 Other Carbohydrate; 2 Vegetables; ½ Fat

---

# Tropical Fruit Curd Decorated with Strawberries in Meringue Pastry Shell

*Traditionally, curds were rich and creamy mixtures made from lemon, lime, or orange juice, thickened and enriched with egg yolks and butter. For a reduced-fat curd with a tropical taste, this recipe calls for naturally dense and rich-tasting sweet mango nectar to be thickened with cornstarch* and flour and then brought to life with a splash of freshly squeezed lime juice, a sprinkle of lime zest, and a pinch of salt.

In Britain, curd is served like jam or jelly as a spread for biscuits and scones. Yet its uses are so much greater. It can be spooned over healthful homestyle cakes, whole grain pancakes and waffles, fresh fruits, or reduced-fat ice creams and low-fat frozen yogurts. Here, it serves as filling for a crisp lime-flavored meringue pastry shell.

YIELD: 9-inch pie with 2⅛ c fruit curd        SERVINGS: 8
SERVING SIZE: 1 wedge (one-eighth pie)

| | WEIGHT | MEASURE |
|---|---|---|
| Lime-Flavored Meringue Pastry Shell (page 174) | | 1 recipe |
| Granulated sugar | 7 oz | 1 c |
| Cornstarch | 1 oz | 3½ tbsp |
| All-purpose flour | | 2 tbsp |
| Salt | | ¼ tsp |
| Mango nectar | | 2 c (1 pt) |
| Fresh lime juice | | 2 tbsp |
| Finely grated lime zest | | 1 tsp |
| Hulled and sliced fresh ripe strawberries | 8 oz | 1⅓ c |

Prepare pastry shell and set aside.

Combine sugar, cornstarch, flour, and salt in a medium saucepan. Mix well. Beating until smooth, slowly add mango nectar. Heat to boiling, then reduce heat to medium. Continue cooking and beating until thick. Remove from heat. Stir in lime juice and zest. Set aside until cool.

Spoon curd into meringue pastry shell. Arrange strawberries over curd. Cut into 8 wedges. Garnish with mint sprigs, if desired, and serve.

---

### NUTRITIONAL FACTS

Calories: 249 (5% from fat)

Fat: 1.6 g (.2 g sat, .6 g mono, .6 g poly)

Protein: 1.8 g and 3%

Carbohydrate: 59.1 g and 92%

Fiber: 1.4 g

Cholesterol: 0 mg

Iron: .5 mg

Sodium: 108.8 mg

Calcium: 15.9 mg

Diabetic Exchanges: ½ Starch; 2 Other Carbohydrates; 1½ Fruits

# Pie Crusts, Tart and Meringue Shells, and Meringue Toppings

Corn Flake Crumb Crust

Crispy Rice Marshmallow Crust

Graham Cracker Crumb Crust

Lemon Marshmallow Meringue Topping

Light and Crisp Phyllo Tart Shells

Lime-Flavored Meringue Pastry Shell

Meringue Topping for Pie

Reduced-Fat and Cholesterol-Free Pastry Crust

Whole Wheat Pastry Crust

# Corn Flake Crumb Crust

*To create this Southwestern-style reduced-fat crumb crust, corn flake crumbs are sweetened with brown sugar and held together with a small amount of melted margarine and apple juice concentrate. It makes the ideal base for Mango Cream Cheese Pie Decorated with Sliced Mangoes (page 154) or Pumpkin Chiffon Pie Dashed with Orange in Corn Flake Crumb Crust (page 159), but can replace the familiar graham cracker crumb crust in a variety of desserts.*

*To make the corn flake crumbs, simply place corn flakes in a heavy plastic bag sealed with the air removed, or between two pieces of plastic wrap or wax paper. Roll over with a rolling pin until fine crumbs form.*

YIELD: 9-inch pie crust
SERVING SIZE: one-eighth pie crust

SERVINGS: 8

|  | WEIGHT | MEASURE |
|---|---|---|
| Butter-flavored vegetable oil cooking spray | — | — |
| Corn flake crumbs | 3 oz | ¾ c |
| Firmly packed light brown sugar | 2 oz | ¼ c |
| Stick margarine, melted | 1 oz | 2 tbsp |
| Thawed apple juice concentrate, undiluted |  | 2 tbsp |

Coat a 9-inch pie pan with cooking spray.

Combine corn flake crumbs and brown sugar in a small bowl. Drizzle melted margarine and juice concentrate over crumb mixture. Mix until crumbs are evenly moistened.

Press evenly into bottom and up sides of prepared pan. If desired, reserve 2 tablespoons crumbs to sprinkle over top of dessert. Refrigerate until use.

---

### NUTRITIONAL FACTS

Calories: 98 (26% from fat)

Fat: 2.9 g (.6 g sat, 1.3 g mono, .9 g poly)

Protein: 1 g and 4%

Carbohydrate: 17.4 g and 70%

Fiber: 0 g

Cholesterol: 0 mg

Iron: 2.8 mg

Sodium: 153.3 mg

Calcium: 8 mg

Diabetic Exchanges: ½ Starch; ½ Other Carbohydrate; ½ Fat

# Crispy Rice
# Marshmallow Crust

*As was the case for most kids from my generation, crispy rice cereal bars were one of my childhood favorites. This recipe takes the fat out of the crunchy bars and transforms them into a pie crust. For an easy-to-make dessert that will appeal to kids of all ages, fill this crust with fat-free frozen yogurt or reduced-fat ice cream and decorate with a complementary fruit sauce and sliced fresh fruit.*

YIELD: 9-inch pie crust                SERVINGS: 8
SERVING SIZE: one-eighth pie crust

|  | WEIGHT | MEASURE |
|---|---|---|
| Butter-flavored vegetable oil cooking spray | — | — |
| Miniature marshmallows | 3 oz | 1½ c |
| Corn syrup | 2 oz | 3 tbsp |
| Granulated sugar | 1 oz | 2 tbsp |
| Oven-toasted rice cereal | 3 oz | 3 c (1½ pt) |

Coat a 9-inch pie pan with cooking spray.

Combine marshmallows, corn syrup, and sugar in a medium saucepan. Cook over low heat, stirring until marshmallows are melted. Remove from heat.

Stir in cereal, mixing until cereal kernels are well coated. Press evenly into bottom and up sides of prepared pan. Refrigerate until chilled and set. Use as directed in recipes such as Strawberry Swirled Vanilla Frozen Yogurt Pie on Crispy Rice Crust (page 201).

---

### NUTRITIONAL FACTS

Calories: 108 (1% from fat)

Fat: .1 g (0 g sat, 0 g mono, .1 g poly)

Protein: .9 g and 3%

Carbohydrate: 26.8 g and 96%

Fiber: .1 g

Cholesterol: 0 mg

Iron: .7 mg

Sodium: 127.6 mg

Calcium: 1.6 mg

Diabetic Exchanges: ½ Starch; 1 Other Carbohydrate

# Graham Cracker Crumb Crust

*Traditionally, graham cracker crusts were prepared from a mixture of cracker crumbs, butter or margarine, and refined white sugar. The crust for an average-size piece of pie yielded about 5 grams of fat. For a healthier version with lots of flavor, the granulated sugar in this recipe is replaced with the richer-tasting brown sugar and the crumbs are moistened and held together with apple juice concentrate and less margarine.*

YIELD: 9-inch pie crust

SERVINGS: 8

SERVING SIZE: one-eighth pie crust

| | WEIGHT | MEASURE |
|---|---|---|
| Butter-flavored vegetable oil cooking spray | — | — |
| Stick margarine | 1½ oz | 3 tbsp |
| Graham cracker crumbs | 6 oz | 1½ c |
| Thawed apple juice concentrate, undiluted | | 2 tbsp |
| Firmly packed light brown sugar | 1 oz | 2 tbsp |

Coat a 9-inch pie pan with cooking spray.

Melt margarine in a small saucepan. Remove from heat. Add cracker crumbs, apple juice concentrate, and brown sugar. Mix until crumbs are evenly moistened. Use your fingers to press crumbs evenly into bottom and up sides of prepared pan.

Refrigerate until chilled and set, or about 1 hour. Use as directed in recipes such as Blackberry Snow Tart in Graham Cracker Crumb Crust (page 142) and Lime Chiffon Angel Pie in Graham Cracker Crumb Crust (page 152).

### VARIATION

Graham Cracker Crumb Crust and Topping: Prepare 1½ recipes Graham Cracker Crumb Crust as directed above. Use ⅔ crumb mixture for crust and the remaining ⅓ crumb mixture to sprinkle on top of pies as directed in recipes such as Banana Lovers' Firm Custard Pie (page 141).

<table>
<tr><td colspan="3" align="center">NUTRITIONAL FACTS</td></tr>
</table>

| | | |
|---|---|---|
| Calories: 144 (40% from fat) | Carbhydrates: 20.4 g and 56% | Sodium: 180.8 mg |
| Fat: 6.4 g (1.2 g sat, 2.8 g mono, 2.2 g poly) | Fiber: .6 g | Calcium: 9.5 mg |
| Protein: 1.5 g and 4% | Cholesterol: 0 mg | Diabetic Exchanges: 1 |
| | Iron: .9 mg | Starch; ½ Fruit; 1 Fat |

# Lemon Marshmallow Meringue Topping

*Eliminating the top pastry crust on a fruit pie can reduce its fat content by one-half and its calories substantially. For a fat-free alternative, cover with a golden brown, soft and puffy meringue. To punch up the taste of the classic whipped egg white topping, this version is sweetened with melted marshmallows and flavored with a splash of freshly squeezed lemon juice and a pinch of finely grated lemon zest.*

YIELD: topping for 9-inch pie          SERVINGS: 8
SERVING SIZE: one-eighth pie topping

| | WEIGHT | MEASURE |
|---|---|---|
| Miniature marshmallows | 7 oz | 3½ c (1¾ pt) |
| Fresh lemon juice | | 2 tbsp |
| Finely grated lemon zest | | 1 tsp |
| Large egg whites, at room temperature | 3¾ oz | 3 |
| Cream of tartar | | ¼ tsp |

Combine marshmallows and lemon juice in a medium saucepan. Cook over medium heat, continually stirring until marshmallows are melted and mixture is smooth. Remove from heat. Stir in lemon zest. Keep warm.

Combine egg whites and cream of tartar in a medium mixing bowl. Beat with an electric mixer until stiff and glossy peaks form.

Fold egg whites into marshmallow mixture. Spread over 9-inch fruit pies such as Peach Pie Topped with Lemon Marshmallow Meringue (page 156). Bake as directed in recipes.

## VARIATION

Orange or Lime Marshmallow Meringue Topping: Replace lemon juice with orange or lime juice and lemon zest with orange or lime zest.

---

### NUTRITIONAL FACTS

| | | |
|---|---|---|
| Calories: 86 (1% from fat) | Fiber: .1 g | Calcium: 2.1 mg |
| Fat: .1 g | Cholesterol: 0 mg | Diabetic Exchanges: |
| Protein: 1.8 g and 8% | Iron: .1 mg | 1½ Other Carbohy- |
| Carbohydrate: 20.7 g and 92% | Sodium: 32.3 mg | drates |

---

# Light and Crisp Phyllo Tart Shells

*Phyllo (pronounced "fee-lo" and sometimes spelled filo or fillo) refers to the tissue-thin sheets of dough used in Greek and Near Eastern dishes such as baklava and spanakopita. Traditionally, sheets of the dough were brushed with melted butter and then stacked or rolled to make pastries with many layers. For a more healthful approach, the dough sheets in these tart shells are sprayed with butter-flavored vegetable oil cooking spray and then brushed with honey before layering in muffin cups.*

*This recipe calls for frozen phyllo dough. It is readily available in most supermarkets in 1-pound packages (about twenty-five sheets). It can be stored in the freezer for up to one year but once thawed it should not be re-frozen because the dough will become brittle. To thaw the dough, place it in the refrigerator overnight or hold it at room temperature for about five hours. Unopened, the phyllo can be stored in the refrigerator for up to one month. Once opened, it should be used within three days. Or use fresh (re-frigerated) phyllo dough if available. It can be found in ethnic markets or specialty-food stores. The fresh dough is easier to work with because the sheets separate more easily than the frozen variety.*

*If this is your first time handling phyllo dough, the instructions on the box are a valuable source of information. These are a few additional tips to assure your success.*

- Set up all tools, cooking containers, and ingredients before opening the dough. Once you begin handling the dough, it is necessary to work quickly.
- Unwrap the dough only when you are ready to begin production. Rewrap any unused dough and refrigerate immediately for future use.
- While working with a sheet of dough, cover remaining sheets with plastic wrap and then a damp towel to avoid drying.
- Work with dry hands to prevent tearing the dough. If it does tear, patch it with some dough from another sheet.

YIELD: 4 tart shells                                        SERVINGS: 4
SERVING SIZE: 1 tart shell

|  | WEIGHT | MEASURE |
|---|---|---|
| Butter-flavored vegetable oil cooking spray |  | 24 one-second sprays |
| Frozen 16½-inch-by-12-inch phyllo dough sheets, thawed |  | 4 sheets |
| Honey, heated until warm |  | 2 tbsp |

Preheat oven to 350 degrees F.

Coat each of 4 muffin cups with a 2-second spray of cooking spray. Carefully unroll dough sheets. Place one dough sheet on a work surface lined with parchment paper. Spray evenly with a 4-second spray of cooking spray. Brush with 1½ teaspoons honey. Cut dough sheet into fourths.

Place 1 dough rectangle coated side up into a muffin cup, gently pressing into bottom and sides of cup. Allow edges to drape over top of cup. Crisscross second dough rectangle over the first one. Repeat twice, crisscrossing 2 more dough rectangles over the previous two. Gently press layer edges together and roll under themselves. Crimp to look like wrinkled tissue paper.

Prick tart shell bottoms with a fork. Bake until golden, or about 10 minutes. Set aside to cool. At serving time, fill tart shells with fruit such as Honey-Glazed Fresh Fruit Melange in Phyllo Tart Shells (page 146) or a curd such as Tropical Fruit Curd Decorated with Strawberries in Meringue Pastry Shell (page 165).

| NUTRITIONAL FACTS | | |
|---|---|---|
| Calories: 126 (35% from fat) | Carbohydrate: 19.4 g and 61% | Sodium: 92.2 mg |
| Fat: 4.9 g (.6 g sat, .6 g mono, .2 g poly) | Fiber: .4 g | Calcium: 2.7 mg |
| Protein: 1.5 g and 5% | Cholesterol: 0 mg | Diabetic Exchanges: 1 Starch; 1 Fat |
| | Iron: .7 mg | |

# Lime-Flavored Meringue Pastry Shell

*Naturally fat-free hard meringues make delightful shells for fruit fillings, curds, chiffons, and low-fat frozen toppings. Prepare extras and store them tightly sealed at room temperature for several days. To redry them completely, place in a 200 degree F oven for 30 minutes.*

YIELD: 9-inch pie crust                                              SERVINGS: 8
SERVING SIZE: one-eighth pie crust

| | WEIGHT | MEASURE |
|---|---|---|
| Butter-flavored vegetable oil cooking spray | — | — |
| Large egg whites, at room temperature | 2½ oz | 2 |
| Fresh lime juice | | 1 tbsp |
| Granulated sugar | 4 oz | ½ c |
| Low-sodium soda cracker crumbs | 1½ oz | ½ c |
| Finely grated lime zest | | 1 tsp |

Preheat oven to 325 degrees F. Coat a 9-inch pie pan with cooking spray.

Combine egg whites and lime juice in a medium mixing bowl. Beat with an electric mixer on high speed until soft peaks form. Continue beating, slowly adding sugar, until stiff peaks form.

Gently fold in cracker crumbs and lime zest. Spread mixture evenly in bottom and up sides of prepared pan. Bake until golden brown, or about

20 minutes. Cool completely on a rack. At serving time, top with filling such as Tropical Fruit Curd Decorated with Strawberries in Meringue Pastry Shell (page 165).

### *VARIATION*

Lemon- or Orange-Flavored Meringue Pastry Shell: Replace lime juice and lime zest with lemon or orange juice and zests.

---

NUTRITIONAL FACTS

Calories: 86 (14% from fat)

Fat: 1.4 g (.2 g sat, .6 g mono, .5 g poly)

Protein: 1.3 g and 6%

Carbohydrate: 17.7 g and 80%

Fiber: .1 g

Cholesterol: 0 mg

Iron: .2 mg

Sodium: 33.7 mg

Calcium: 7.5 mg

Diabetic Exchanges: ½ Starch; ½ Other Carbohydrate; ½ Fat

---

# Meringue Topping for Pie

*When I was a young baker, my mother always assured me that the meringue topping on my pies puddled because of the humid weather. In reality, the cause was more likely that I had spread the meringue over a cool or lukewarm filling. When placed in the oven, the top of the meringue became piping hot and cooked while the bottom remained undercooked. As the meringue stood, the egg whites lost moisture and leaked. Now I know that spreading the meringue over a hot filling will prevent it from weeping. The heat of the filling will cook the bottom of the meringue.*

YIELD: topping for 9-inch pie

SERVINGS: one-eighth pie topping

SERVINGS: 8

| | WEIGHT | MEASURE |
|---|---|---|
| Large egg whites, at room temperature | 2½ oz | 2 |
| Cream of tartar | | ¼ tsp |
| Sifted powdered sugar | 1 oz | ¼ c |
| Vanilla extract | | ½ tsp |

Combine egg whites and cream of tartar in a medium mixing bowl. Beat with an electric mixer until soft peaks form. Continue beating, adding powdered sugar 1 tablespoon at a time until stiff, glossy peaks form. Fold in vanilla.

Spread meringue over pies such as Pineapple Custard Cream Meringue Pie (page 158) or Lemon Meringue Pie in Whole Wheat Crust (page 151). Seal meringue to pastry shell to prevent shrinkage. Bake as directed in recipes.

---

### NUTRITIONAL FACTS

| | | |
|---|---|---|
| Calories: 19 (0% from fat) | Fiber: 0 g | Calcium: .6 mg |
| Fat: 0 g | Cholesterol: 0 mg | Diabetic Exchanges: Free |
| Protein: .9 g and 19% | Iron: 0 mg | Food |
| Carbohydrate: 3.7 g and 81% | Sodium: 13.8 mg | |

# Reduced-Fat and Cholesterol-Free Pastry Crust

*As with higher-fat pastry crusts, this pie dough should be kept cool during mixing and handling. For best results, chill the dough to 50 to 60 degrees F before rolling. This will allow the water and fruit juice concentrate to distribute evenly throughout the dough and harden the margarine so that it won't soften during rolling.*

YIELD: two 9-inch pie crusts and cutouts for tops     SERVINGS: 16
SERVING SIZE: one-eighth pie crust and top cutouts

| | WEIGHT | MEASURE |
|---|---|---|
| All-purpose flour | 10½ oz | 2⅓ c (1⅙ pt) |
| Baking powder | | ½ tsp |
| Salt | | ½ tsp |
| Stick margarine, chilled | 4 oz | ½ c |
| Thawed white grape juice concentrate, undiluted | | 3 tbsp |
| Very cold water | | 2 to 3 tbsp |

Combine flour, baking powder, and salt in a medium bowl. Mix well. Cut margarine into flour with a pastry blender or two knives until mixture resembles coarse crumbs. Slowly add grape juice concentrate and water, tossing with a fork until flour is moistened without being wet.

Divide dough into 2 equal parts. Remove ⅓ dough from each half. Gently press the 4 dough pieces between 2 sheets of wax paper or parchment paper into four flattened rounds. Chill at least 30 minutes or up to an hour for ease in handling.

Roll each large dough piece with a rolling pin between 2 sheets of wax paper or parchment paper or on a lightly floured work surface into 10½-inch rounds of even thickness (about ⅛ inch).

Fit each 10½-inch dough round into a 9-inch pie pan. Fold edges over pans and flute crusts if desired.

Roll small dough pieces between 2 sheets of wax paper or parchment paper or on a lightly floured work surface into rounds of even thickness (about ⅛ inch). Remove top sheet of paper. Cut dough with small cutters into decorative shapes.

Pour pie filling such as Red Cherry Pie Splashed with Amaretto (page 161) into crust. Arrange decorative cutouts on top. Bake as directed in recipe.

## NUTRITIONAL FACTS

| | | |
|---|---|---|
| Calories: 125 (43% from fat) | Carbohydrate: 15.8 g and 51% | Sodium: 147.4 mg |
| | | Calcium: 5.4 mg |
| Fat: 5.9 g (1.2 g sat, 2.6 g mono, 1.9 g poly) | Fiber: .5 g | Diabetic Exchanges: 1 Starch; 1 Fat |
| | Cholesterol: 0 mg | |
| Protein: 2 g and 6% | Iron: .9 mg | |

# Whole Wheat Pastry Crust

*Traditional pie crusts are made with one-half cup or more of butter, lard, or shortening per crust. This crust not only contains half the traditional crust's fat but the fat of choice is polyunsaturated margarine. Another bonus: This crust is made with vitamin- and fiber-rich whole wheat flour.*

*A splash of almond extract and a sprinkle of sugar round out the crust's hearty whole grain flavor.*

YIELD: 9-inch pie crust                                    SERVINGS: 8
SERVING SIZE: one-eighth crust

|  | WEIGHT | MEASURE |
|---|---|---|
| Whole wheat pastry flour or whole wheat flour | 4 oz | scant 1 c |
| Granulated sugar |  | 2 tsp |
| Salt |  | ¼ tsp |
| Baking powder |  | ¼ tsp |
| Stick margarine, chilled | 2 oz | ¼ c |
| Very cold water |  | 1½ tbsp |
| Distilled vinegar |  | 2 tsp |
| Almond extract |  | ¼ tsp |

Combine flour, sugar, salt, and baking powder in a small bowl. Mix well. Cut margarine into flour with a pastry blender or two knives until mixture resembles coarse crumbs.

Slowly add water, vinegar, and almond extract, tossing with a fork until flour is moistened without being wet. If mixture seems dry or crumbly, sprinkle in 1 teaspoon cold water. The dough should not be damp or sticky.

Gently press dough into a flattened round. Chill at least 30 minutes for ease in handling.

Roll dough with a rolling pin between two sheets of parchment paper or wax paper or on a lightly floured work surface into 10½-inch round of even thickness (about ⅛ inch). Fit dough round into a 9-inch pie pan. Fold edges over pan and flute crust, if desired.

For unbaked crust: Do not prick crust. Pour fillings such as Honey-Sweetened Sweet Potato Pie with a Splash of Bourbon Whiskey (page 147) and Apple Pie Just Like Grandma's (page 140) into crust. Bake as directed in recipes.

For baked crust: With a fork, lightly prick crust's bottom, sides, and where sides and bottom meet. Bake in 400 degree F oven until golden brown, or about 10 minutes. Use as directed in recipes for pies such as Lemon Meringue Pie in Whole Wheat Crust (page 151).

## NUTRITIONAL FACTS

Calories: 103 (49% from fat)

Fat: 5.9 g (1.1 g sat, 2.5 g mono, 1.8 g poly)

Protein: 2 g and 7%

Carbohydrate: 11.5 g and 43%

Fiber: 1.4 g

Cholesterol: 0 mg

Iron: .5 mg

Sodium: 146.8 mg

Calcium: 11.7 mg

Diabetic Exchanges: ½ Starch; ½ Other Carbohydrate; 1 Fat

# Frozen Yogurts, Sherbets, Ice Creams, Sorbets, and Other Frozen Desserts

Baked Banana and Marshmallow Sundae with Strawberry Jam

Banana and Strawberry Low-Fat Frozen Yogurt

Chunky Pineapple Buttermilk Sherbet

Creamy Banana and Peach Sherbet

Dried Plum (Prune) and Raspberry Sorbet

Frozen Pumpkin Ice Cream Dessert
with Gingersnap Crumb Crust

Honey-Flavored Mango and Ginger Frozen Yogurt

Orange Fat-Free and Sugar-Free Sherbet

Peach and Strawberry Frozen Yogurt

Pina Colada Reduced-Fat Ice Cream

Pumpkin Pie Fat-Free Ice Cream

Rum Raisin Low-Fat Ice Cream

Strawberry Amaretto Glacé

Strawberry Cheesecake Fat-Free Ice Cream

Strawberry Swirled Vanilla Frozen Yogurt Pie
on Crispy Rice Crust

# Baked Banana and Marshmallow Sundae with Strawberry Jam

*These sundaes are more than a scoop of ice cream topped with a sweet sauce, a sprinkle of chopped nuts, and a squirt of whipped cream. Miniature marshmallows are sandwiched between ripe, sweet banana halves and then baked in parchment paper packages. After cutting the packages open to display the steaming and fragrant bananas with melted marshmallows, the fruit is topped with a scoop of vanilla frozen yogurt and a drizzle of warm strawberry spread. These sundaes are large enough to share, so plan that this recipe will serve eight diners rather than the four listed unless guests are very hungry.*

YIELD: 4 sundaes
SERVING SIZE: 1 banana, ½ c frozen yogurt, and 2 tbsp topping

|  | WEIGHT | MEASURE |
| --- | --- | --- |
| Parchment paper |  | 4 sheets |
| Ripe bananas, peeled | 20 oz as purchased | 4 small |
| Miniature marshmallows | 3 oz | 1½ c |
| Butter-flavored vegetable oil cooking spray | — | — |
| Vanilla fat-free frozen yogurt | 12 oz | 2 c (1 pt) |
| 100%-fruit strawberry spread, melted | 5½ oz | ½ c |

Cut parchment paper into 4 heart shapes large enough to hold a banana and still have room for crimping edges. Preheat oven to 450 degrees F.

Slice bananas in half lengthwise. Place one sliced banana on one side of each heart. Spoon about ¾ ounce (6 tablespoons) marshmallows between banana halves.

Seal packages by folding empty half of parchment paper over each banana. Then, starting at top of fold, make a small crimp in edge. Continue crimping around edge. Each crimp should hold the previous one in place. When bottom of heart is reached, fold point under to hold in place. Coat parchment packages with cooking spray. Place on a baking tray. Bake until parchment is puffed and brown, or about 10 minutes.

Place packages on 4 dessert plates and cut them open to display bananas and release their aromas. Top each with a 3-ounce (½-cup) scoop of frozen yogurt and drizzle each with 1½ ounces (2 tablespoons) of melted strawberry spread.

---

### NUTRITIONAL FACTS

Calories: 436 (1% from fat)

Fat: .7 g (.3 g sat, .1 g mono, .1 g poly)

Protein: 6.1 g and 5%

Carbohydrate: 106.2 g and 93%

Fiber: 2.5 g

Cholesterol: 1.3 mg

Iron: .8 mg

Sodium: 79.7 mg

Calcium: 162.1 mg

Diabetic Exchanges: ½ Starch; 4 Other Carbohydrates; 2 Fruits; ½ Skim Milk

---

# Banana and Strawberry Low-Fat Frozen Yogurt

*Did you know that botanically, bananas are berries? They are classified in this manner because they are simple fruits with pulpy or fleshy pericarps (the walls of a mature ovary), having one or more seeds in the flesh but no true stones.*

YIELD: 2½ c (1¼ pt) frozen yogurt

SERVING SIZE: ½ c frozen yogurt

SERVINGS: 5

|  | WEIGHT | MEASURE |
|---|---|---|
| Very ripe banana, peeled and sliced thick | 6 oz | 1 medium |
| Fresh ripe or frozen unsweetened strawberries | 6 oz | 1 c |
| Fat-free plain yogurt | 9 oz | 1 c |
| Thawed white grape juice concentrate, undiluted |  | ¼ c + 2 tbsp |
| Vanilla extract |  | ½ tsp |

Combine all ingredients except sliced strawberries in a food processor or blender. Blend until smooth. Pour mixture into freezer container of an ice cream freezer. Freeze according to manufacturer's instructions. Serve immediately, or spoon into a covered airtight container and freeze.

Alternatively, to still-freeze frozen yogurt, pour ¼-inch layer of mixture into a nonreactive metal pan. Cover tightly and freeze until almost firm.

Break into small chunks with a heavy spoon. Process briefly in a food processor or blender, or beat in a mixing bowl until just slushy, beginning with mixer on low speed and increasing to medium as mixture softens.

Repeat freezing and beating 3 times at half-hour intervals. Serve after final beating or freeze until serving time. If frozen yogurt is frozen hard, place in refrigerator until slightly softened, or 15 to 20 minutes, before scooping. Scoop into 5 dessert dishes. Garnish each with hulled strawberry slices, if desired, and serve.

### NUTRITIONAL FACTS

| | | |
|---|---|---|
| Calories: 109 (4% from fat) | Carbohydrate: 23.9 g and 84% | Sodium: 41.5 mg |
| Fat: .5g (.2 g sat, .1 g mono, .1 g poly) | Fiber: 1.7 g | Calcium: 111.2 mg |
| Protein: 3.6 g and 13% | Cholesterol: 1 mg | Diabetic Exchanges: 1 Fruit; ½ Skim Milk |
| | Iron: .4 mg | |

# Chunky Pineapple Buttermilk Sherbet

*Growing up, I always looked forward to my mother's homemade sherbets. This recipe is an adaptation of her pineapple sherbet. It requires only three ingredients. Buttermilk's creamy consistency and hint of tartness balances a mixture of intensely flavored sweet pineapple juice concentrate and chunky-textured crushed pineapple.*

YIELD: 4 c (1 qt) sherbet
SERVING SIZE: ½ cup sherbet

SERVINGS: 8

|  | WEIGHT | MEASURE |
|---|---|---|
| Low-fat buttermilk |  | 2 c (1 pt) |
| Drained crushed pineapple canned in juice | 9 oz | 1 c |
| Thawed pineapple juice concentrate, undiluted |  | ¾ c |

Combine all ingredients in a bowl. Mix until well blended. Pour mixture into freezer container of an ice cream freezer and freeze according to manufacturer's instructions. Serve immediately, or spoon into a covered airtight container and freeze.

Alternatively, to still-freeze sherbet, pour ¼-inch layer of mixture into a nonreactive metal pan. Cover tightly and freeze until almost firm.

Break into small chunks with a heavy spoon. Beat in a mixing bowl until just slushy, beginning with mixer on low speed and increasing to medium as mixture softens.

Repeat freezing and beating 3 times at half-hour intervals. Serve after final beating or freeze until serving time. If sherbet is frozen hard, place in refrigerator until slightly softened, or 15 to 20 minutes, before scooping. Scoop into 8 dessert dishes and serve.

---

### NUTRITIONAL FACTS

Calories: 67 (3% from fat)
Fat: .3 g (.1 g sat, 0 g mono, .1 g poly)
Protein: .8 g and 4%

Carbohydrate: 16.3 g and 92%
Fiber: .6 g
Cholesterol: .5 mg
Iron: .4 mg

Sodium: 11.3 mg
Calcium: 16.7 mg
Diabetic Exchanges: 1 Fruit

---

# Creamy Banana and Peach Sherbet

*A purée of potassium-rich ripe, sweet bananas gives this low-fat frozen sherbet the creamy texture of ice cream without its fat, sugar, or calories. When purchasing bananas, keep in mind that they are harvested and shipped green. As they ripen they turn yellow. Brown spots appear naturally and usually do not affect the fruits' quality. Once ripe, bananas may be refrigerated for a day or so. Their flesh color and quality won't be hindered but their skin will turn black.*

YIELD: 8 c (2 qt) sherbet          SERVINGS: 16
SERVING SIZE: ½ c sherbet

| | WEIGHT | MEASURE |
|---|---|---|
| Peeled fresh ripe peach slices or sliced frozen unsweetened peaches | 1¼ lb | 3⅓ c (1⅔ pt) |
| Peeled ripe banana slices | 8 oz | 1½ c |
| Low-fat milk | | 2 c (1 pt) |
| Thawed white grape juice concentrate, undiluted | | ¾ c |

Peel peaches by blanching in boiling water for 20 to 60 seconds and then placing them in ice water or under cold running water until completely cooled. The skins should slip off easily.

Combine peaches, bananas, milk, and grape juice concentrate in a food processor or blender. Blend until smooth. Pour mixture into freezer container of an ice cream freezer. Freeze according to manufacturer's instructions. Serve immediately, or spoon into a covered airtight container and freeze.

Alternatively, to still-freeze sherbet, pour ¼-inch layer of mixture into a nonreactive metal pan. Cover tightly and freeze until almost firm.

Break into small chunks with a heavy spoon. Process briefly in a food processor or blender, or beat in a mixing bowl, until just slushy, beginning with mixer on low speed and increasing to medium as mixture softens.

Repeat freezing and beating 3 times at half-hour intervals. Serve after final beating or freeze until serving time. If sherbet is frozen hard, place in refrigerator until slightly softened, or 15 to 20 minutes, before scooping. Scoop into 16 dessert dishes. Garnish each with 2 peeled peach slices, if desired, and serve.

# Dried Plum (Prune) and Raspberry Sorbet

*A sorbet is understood to be a purée of fruits or vegetables. This fruit sorbet meets this criteria but fortunately does not contain the sugar traditionally used to create the smooth texture characteristic of these frozen flavored ices. Since this deep reddish-brown sorbet is sweetened with fruit juice concentrate, it relies on the rich and full body of dried plum and raspberry purées along with quick, even freezing to yield a pleasing mouthfeel. As for other sorbets, the sweetened fruit purée for this fruit ice should taste very strong and very sweet before freezing. Then, once frozen, it will taste just right. For maximum texture and flavor, serve this and other sorbets at soft-serve consistency.*

YIELD: 3 c (1½ pt) sorbet                    SERVINGS: 6
SERVING SIZE: ½ c sorbet

|  | WEIGHT | MEASURE |
|---|---|---|
| Frozen unsweetened or fresh raspberries | 4½ oz | 1 c |
| Prune purée (page 5) or prune baby food | 5 oz | ½ c + 2 tbsp |
| Thawed white grape juice concentrate, undiluted |  | ½ c |
| Water |  | 1½ c |

Place raspberries in a blender or food processor. Blend until smooth. Strain through a fine mesh strainer (to remove seeds) into a bowl. Add prune purée, grape juice concentrate, and water. Mix until smooth. Pour mixture into freezer container of an ice cream freezer. Freeze according to manufacturer's instructions. Serve immediately, or spoon into a covered airtight container and freeze.

Alternatively, to still-freeze sorbet, pour ¼-inch layer of mixture into a nonreactive metal pan. Cover tightly and freeze until almost firm.

Break into small chunks with a heavy spoon. Process briefly in a food processor or blender, or beat in a mixing bowl until just slushy, beginning with mixer on low speed and increasing to medium as mixture softens.

Repeat freezing and beating 3 times at half-hour intervals. Serve after final beating or freeze until serving time. If sorbet is frozen hard, place in refrigerator until slightly softened, or 15 to 20 minutes, before scooping. Scoop into 6 dessert dishes. Garnish each dish with 1 tablespoon raspberries and a mint sprig, if desired, and serve.

---

### NUTRITIONAL FACTS

Calories: 114 (2% from fat)
Fat: .2 g (0 g sat, 0 g mono, .1 g poly)
Protein: .9 g and 3%

Carbohydrate: 28.5 g and 95%
Fiber: 2.3 g
Cholesterol: 0 mg
Iron: .9 mg

Sodium: 8.9 mg
Calcium: 16.3 mg
Diabetic Exchanges: 2 Fruits

---

# Frozen Pumpkin Ice Cream Dessert with Gingersnap Crumb Crust

*In addition to its tantalizing taste and vibrant color, pumpkin is rich in nutrients, especially beta-carotene. Blended with vanilla low-fat ice cream and sweet spices and then sandwiched between gingersnap crumb crusts, this pumpkin dessert is not just for Halloween and Thanksgiving.*

YIELD: 13-by-9-inch dessert

SERVINGS: 24

SERVING SIZE: 2⅛-by-2¼-inch piece

| | WEIGHT | MEASURE |
|---|---|---|
| Butter-flavored vegetable oil cooking spray | — | — |
| Gingersnap crumbs | 10½ oz | 2⅔ c (1⅓ pt) |
| Stick margarine, melted | 1½ oz | 3 tbsp |
| Vanilla low-fat ice cream, softened | 3 lb | 2 qt |
| Canned pumpkin | 9 oz | 1 c |
| Firmly packed light brown sugar | 8 oz | 1 c |
| Ground cinnamon | | 1 tsp |
| Ground ginger | | ½ tsp |
| Ground allspice | | ¼ tsp |
| Ground cloves | | ⅛ tsp |

Coat a 13-by-9-by-2-inch baking pan with cooking spray.

Combine gingersnap crumbs and melted margarine in a medium bowl. Mix well.

Combine ice cream, pumpkin, brown sugar, cinnamon, ginger, allspice, and cloves in a large bowl. Whisk until well blended.

Pat one-half gingersnap crumb mixture into prepared pan. Spread pumpkin mixture evenly over gingersnap crust. Sprinkle remaining gingersnap crumbs evenly over top.

Freeze until firm. Cut into 24 pieces and serve.

## NUTRITIONAL FACTS

Calories: 177 (20% from fat)

Fat: 4 g (.9 g sat, 1.3 g mono, .6 g poly)

Protein: 2.8 g and 6%

Carbohydrate: 33.3 g and 74%

Fiber: 1.2 g

Cholesterol: 3.3 mg

Iron: 1.1 mg

Sodium: 150.8 mg

Calcium: 88.2 mg

Diabetic Exchanges: 2 Other Carbohydrates; ½ Low-Fat Milk

# Honey-Flavored Mango and Ginger Frozen Yogurt

*One taste of this honey-sweetened, creamy mango-flavored frozen yogurt laced with bits of crystallized ginger and you'll know why mangoes are rated the world's most popular fruit. While previously rare in supermarkets throughout the United States, this nutrient-rich tropical fruit with its peachlike flavor is now readily available nationwide.*

YIELD: 6 c (1½ qt) frozen yogurt  
SERVING SIZE: ½ c frozen yogurt

SERVINGS: 12

|  | WEIGHT | MEASURE |
|---|---|---|
| Fat-free plain yogurt | 34 oz | 4 c (1 qt) |
| Puréed mango (about 2 medium) | 10 oz | 1¼ c |
| Honey | 9 oz | ¾ c |
| Finely chopped crystallized ginger | 1 oz | 2 tbsp |

Combine yogurt, mango purée, and honey in a medium bowl. Whisk until well blended.

Pour mixture into freezer container of an ice cream freezer. Freeze according to manufacturer's instructions. When partially frozen, mix in ginger. When frozen, serve immediately, or spoon into a covered airtight container and freeze.

Alternatively, to still-freeze yogurt, pour ¼-inch layer of mixture (without ginger) into a nonreactive metal pan. Cover tightly and freeze until almost firm.

Break into small chunks with a heavy spoon. Process briefly in a food processor or blender, or beat in a mixing bowl until just slushy, beginning mixer on low speed and increasing to medium as mixture softens.

Repeat freezing and beating 3 times at half-hour intervals. After final beating, mix in ginger. Serve or freeze until serving time. If yogurt is frozen hard, place in refrigerator until slightly softened, or 15 to 20 minutes, before scooping. Scoop into 12 dessert dishes and serve.

## NUTRITIONAL FACTS

Calories: 155 (2% from fat)

Fat: .3 g (.1 g sat, .1 g mono, 0 g poly)

Protein: 5 g and 12%

Carbohydrate: 35.4 g and 86%

Fiber: 1.1 g

Cholesterol: 1.6 mg

Iron: .3 mg

Sodium: 65.7 mg

Calcium: 172.6 mg

Diabetic Exchanges: 1 Other Carbohydrate; 1 Fruit; ½ Skim Milk

# Orange Fat-Free and Sugar-Free Sherbet

*This recipe is an adaptation of another one of my mother's recipes. When she was in the mood for healthy orange sherbet, she would mix frozen orange juice concentrate with skim milk and freeze it in a metal ice cube tray. Every half hour or so for the next few hours she would pull out the frozen mixture and stir it until just slushy. This recipe is nearly the same as my mom's, but fat-free half-and-half replaces the skim milk for a richer, creamier taste.*

YIELD: 2½ c (1¼ pt) sherbet          SERVINGS: 5
SERVING SIZE: ½ c sherbet

| | WEIGHT | MEASURE |
|---|---|---|
| Thawed orange juice concentrate, undiluted | | ½ c + 2 tbsp |
| Fat-free half-and-half | | 2 c (1 pt) |

Combine orange juice concentrate and half-and-half in a medium bowl. Mix until well blended. Pour mixture into freezer container of an ice cream freezer. Freeze according to manufacturer's instructions. Serve immediately, or spoon into a covered airtight container and freeze.

Alternatively, to still-freeze sherbet, pour ¼-inch layer of mixture into a nonreactive metal pan. Cover tightly and freeze until almost firm.

Break into small chunks with a heavy spoon. Process briefly in a food processor or blender, or beat in a mixing bowl until just slushy, beginning mixer on low and increasing to medium speed as mixture softens.

Repeat freezing and beating 3 times at half-hour intervals. Serve after final beating or freeze until serving time. If sherbet is frozen hard, place in refrigerator until slightly softened, or 15 to 20 minutes, before scooping. Scoop into 5 dessert dishes. Garnish with orange knots, if desired, and serve. To create orange knots, cut a thin slice from each end of an orange with a small, sharp, pointed knife. Stand orange on end. With the knife tip, cut peel from top to bottom in long thin strips. Tie each strip into a knot, being careful not to break it. Use the peeled fruit for fresh juice, or cut into sections or thin rounds and use to decorate the orange sherbet along with the orange knots.

Instead of in a dish, offer this sherbet in a hollowed-out frozen orange shell, if desired. Simply slice ½ inch from the top of the orange to prevent the shell from toppling over, cut a thin slice of peel from the bottom, and scoop out the fruit and freeze the shell.

---

### NUTRITIONAL FACTS

Calories: 98 (0% from fat)     Fiber:—g                          Calcium:—mg
Fat: 0 g                                 Cholesterol: 0 mg          Diabetic Exchanges: 1
Protein: 3.9 g and 20%         Iron:—mg                         Fruit; ½ Skim Milk
Carbohydrate: 16.2 g and     Sodium: 98.6 mg
   80%

---

# Peach and Strawberry Frozen Yogurt

*There are many reasons to eat produce. It contains no saturated fat, little sodium, lots of fiber, and generous amounts of antioxidant vitamins. Now,* Tufts University Health & Nutrition Letter *has reported that scientists from the United Kingdom are examining yet another component of produce: salicylic acid. Salicylic acid is one of the active ingredients in aspirin. While the amounts of salicylates in food are much less than those in aspirin, they may stem inflammation in the blood vessels that could otherwise lead to hardening of the arteries. Berries, cherries, oranges, and peppers are particularly good sources of salicylates. (Many spices contain salicylates, too.)*

*So if you need another reason to try this creamy fruit juice–sweetened frozen yogurt flavored with peaches as well as both fresh strawberries and strawberry spread, now you've got it.*

YIELD: 4½ c (1⅛ qt) frozen yogurt          SERVINGS: 9
SERVING SIZE: ½ c frozen yogurt

|  | WEIGHT | MEASURE |
|---|---|---|
| Unflavored gelatin |  | 1 tsp |
| Thawed white grape juice concentrate, undiluted |  | ¼ c + 2 tbsp |
| Peeled and sliced fresh ripe peaches or frozen unsweetened peaches | 22 oz | 3½ c (4 medium) |
| Hulled fresh ripe or frozen unsweetened strawberries | 12 oz | 2 c (1 pt) |
| 100%-fruit strawberry spread | 5 oz | scant ½ c |
| Fat-free plain yogurt | 9 oz | 1 c |
| Almond extract |  | ½ tsp |

Sprinkle gelatin over grape juice concentrate in a small saucepan. Let stand until it swells to a spongy consistency, or about 5 minutes. Place over low heat, stirring until gelatin is completely dissolved. Cool.

Peel the peaches by blanching in boiling water for 20 to 60 seconds, and then placing them in ice water or under cold running water until completely cooled. The skins should slip off easily.

Combine peaches, strawberries, and strawberry spread in a food processor or blender. Blend until smooth. Add yogurt, almond extract, and gelatin mixture to the blender or food processor. Blend until smooth. Pour mixture into freezer container of an ice cream freezer. Freeze according to manufacturer's instructions. Serve immediately, or spoon into a covered airtight container and freeze.

Alternatively, to still-freeze yogurt, pour ¼-inch layer of mixture into a nonreactive metal pan. Cover tightly and freeze until almost firm.

Break into small chunks with a heavy spoon. Process briefly in a food processor or blender, or beat in a mixing bowl until just slushy, beginning with mixer on low speed and increasing to medium as mixture softens.

Repeat freezing and beating 3 times at half-hour intervals. Serve after final beating or freeze until serving time. If yogurt is frozen hard, place in refrigerator until slightly softened, or 15 to 20 minutes, before scooping. Scoop into 9 dessert dishes and serve.

NUTRITIONAL FACTS

| | | |
|---|---|---|
| Calories: 102 (2% from fat) | Carbohydrate: 23 g and 87% | Iron: .3 mg |
| Fat: .3 g (.1 g sat, .1 g mono, .1 g poly) | Alcohol: .2 g and 1% | Sodium: 26.4 mg |
| Protein: 2.6 g and 10% | Fiber: 1.8 g | Calcium: 65.6 mg |
| | Cholesterol: .6 mg | Diabetic Exchanges: 1 Fruit; ½ Skim Milk |

# Pina Colada Reduced-Fat Ice Cream

*A pina colada is a tropical drink made from coconut cream, pineapple juice, and rum, served over ice and garnished with a pineapple chunk. This fruit juice–sweetened and reduced-fat creamy frozen version of the cocktail is prepared by blending pineapple chunks with white grape and pineapple juice concentrates, light coconut milk, and rum extract and then freezing.*

YIELD: 4 c (1 qt) ice cream
SERVING SIZE: ½ c ice cream

SERVINGS: 8

| | WEIGHT | MEASURE |
|---|---|---|
| Pineapple chunks canned in juice | 8-oz can | |
| Light coconut milk | 14-oz can | 1¾ c |
| Thawed pineapple juice concentrate, undiluted | | ½ c |
| Thawed white grape juice concentrate, undiluted | | ¼ c + 1 tbsp |
| Rum extract | | 1 tsp |
| Pure coconut extract | | ¼ tsp |

Empty one 8-ounce can pineapple chunks with its juice into a blender or food processor. Blend until smooth. Add coconut milk, juice concentrates, and extracts. Mix until well blended. Pour mixture into freezer container of an ice cream freezer. Freeze according to manufacturer's instructions. Serve immediately, or spoon into a covered airtight container and freeze.

Alternatively, to still-freeze ice cream, pour ¼-inch layer of mixture into a nonreactive metal pan. Cover tightly and freeze until almost firm.

Break into small chunks with a heavy spoon. Process briefly in a food processor or blender, or beat in a mixing bowl until just slushy, beginning with mixer on low speed and increasing to medium as mixture softens.

Repeat freezing and beating 3 times at half-hour intervals. Serve after final beating or freeze until serving time. If ice cream is frozen hard, place in refrigerator until slightly softened, or 15 to 20 minutes, before scooping. Scoop into 8 dessert dishes. Garnish with pineapple chunks, if desired, and serve.

---

### NUTRITIONAL FACTS

Calories: 95 (24% from fat)
Fat: 2.7 g (1.6 g sat, 0 g mono, 0 g poly)
Protein: 1 g and 4%

Carbohydrate: 17.7 g and 70%
Alcohol: .4 g and 3%
Fiber: .4 g
Cholesterol: 0 mg

Iron: .3 mg
Sodium: 14.4 mg
Calcium: 11 mg
Diabetic Exchanges: 1 Fruit; ½ Fat

---

# Pumpkin Pie Fat-Free Ice Cream

*For those who believe that if you take the fat out of ice cream it is never going to taste as good as the regular stuff, this recipe is a must try. It's easy to make, besides. Canned pumpkin is blended with fat-free half-and-half and maple syrup, then seasoned with cinnamon, ginger, and nutmeg, and frozen. A taste of the creamy, sweet dessert is sure to get you reminiscing about Thanksgiving.*

YIELD: 7½ c (scant 2 qt) ice cream          SERVINGS: 15
SERVING SIZE: ½ c ice cream

|  | WEIGHT | MEASURE |
|---|---|---|
| Fat-free half-and-half |  | 4 c (1 qt) |
| Canned pumpkin | 15-oz can | 1⅔ c |
| Maple syrup | 14 oz | 1¼ c |
| Ground cinnamon |  | 1 tsp |
| Ground ginger |  | ½ tsp |
| Ground nutmeg |  | ¼ tsp |

Combine all ingredients in a large bowl. Whisk until well blended. Pour mixture into freezer container of an ice cream freezer. Freeze according to manufacturer's instructions. Serve immediately, or spoon into a covered airtight container and freeze.

Alternatively, to still-freeze ice cream, pour a ¼-inch layer of mixture into a nonreactive metal pan. Cover tightly and freeze until almost firm.

Break into small chunks with a heavy spoon. Process briefly in a food processor or blender, or beat in a mixing bowl until just slushy, beginning with mixer on low speed and increasing to medium as mixture softens.

Repeat freezing and beating 3 times at half-hour intervals. Serve after final beating or freeze until serving time. If ice cream is frozen hard, place in refrigerator until slightly softened, or 15 to 20 minutes, before scooping. Scoop into 15 dessert dishes and serve.

NUTRITIONAL FACTS

| | | |
|---|---|---|
| Calories: 122 (1% from fat) | Carbohydrate: 26.7 g and 91% | Sodium: 56.5 mg |
| Fat: .2 g (.1 g sat, 0 g mono, 0 g poly) | Fiber: .9 g | Calcium: 27.3 mg |
| Protein: 2.4 g and 8% | Cholesterol: 0 mg | Diabetic Exchanges: 1 |
| | Iron: .8 mg | Other Carbohydrate; |
| | | ½ Fruit; ½ Skim Milk |

# Rum Raisin Low-Fat Ice Cream

*Rum raisin ice cream was one of my favorite desserts until I discovered the amount of fat, cholesterol, and calories in a mere cup of my preferred brand. This reduced-fat version is creamy and rich with only half the fat, cholesterol, and calories. Its secret is custard thickened with cornstarch and then blended with marshmallow creme, a splash of rum extract, and plump seedless raisins.*

YIELD: 4 c (1 qt) ice cream            SERVINGS: 8
SERVING SIZE: ½ c ice cream

| | WEIGHT | MEASURE |
|---|---|---|
| Cornstarch | 1 oz | 3½ tbsp |
| Honey | | 3 tbsp |
| Low-fat milk, heated | | 3 c (1½ pt) |
| Marshmallow creme | 4 oz | 1¼ c |
| Rum extract | | 1 tsp |
| Firmly packed raisins | 3 oz | ½ c |

Combine cornstarch and honey in a medium saucepan. Mix until blended. Gradually beat in hot milk. Beating constantly, heat to a boil. Reduce heat and simmer until thickened, or about 3 minutes.

Transfer mixture to a storage container. Place a sheet of parchment or wax paper on top of mixture to prevent a skin from forming. Refrigerate until no longer warm.

Combine milk mixture, marshmallow creme, and rum extract in a blender or food processor. Blend until smooth. Pour mixture into freezer container of an ice cream freezer. Freeze according to manufacturer's instructions. When partially frozen, mix in raisins. When frozen, serve or spoon into a covered airtight container and freeze.

Alternatively, to still-freeze ice cream, pour ¼-inch layer of mixture (without raisins) into a nonreactive metal pan. Cover tightly and freeze until almost firm.

Break into small chunks with a heavy spoon. Process briefly in a food processor or blender, or beat in a mixing bowl until just slushy, beginning with mixer on low speed and increasing to medium as mixture softens.

Repeat freezing and beating 3 times at half-hour intervals. After beating third time, mix in raisins. Serve or freeze until serving time. If ice cream is frozen hard, place in refrigerator until slightly softened, or 15 to 20 minutes, before scooping. Scoop into 8 dessert dishes and serve.

---

### NUTRITIONAL FACTS

| | | |
|---|---|---|
| Calories: 158 (6% from fat) | Carbohydrate: 34.4 g and 84% | Sodium: 59.9 mg |
| Fat: 1 g (.6 g sat, .3 g mono, .1 g poly) | Alcohol: .4 g and 2% | Calcium: 118.3 mg |
| | Fiber: .5 g | Diabetic Exchanges: 1½ |
| Protein: 3.4 g and 8% | Cholesterol: 3.7 mg | Other Carbohydrates; |
| | Iron: .3 mg | ½ Fruit; ½ Skim Milk |

---

# Strawberry Amaretto Glacé

*Glacé (glahs-say) is the French word for iced or frozen. Offer this luscious low-fat and vitamin C–rich glacé as an intermezzo or final course in a special meal. The fruit juice–sweetened and amaretto-flavored fruit ice will cleanse yet tantalize the palate. For a sophisticated yet easy-to-make dessert, serve a scoop of this bright red strawberry glacé on a slice of angel food cake or in a crisp meringue shell, sprinkle with sliced berries, and drizzle with amaretto.*

YIELD: 4 c (1 qt) glacé
SERVING SIZE: ½ c glacé

SERVINGS: 8

| | WEIGHT | MEASURE |
|---|---|---|
| Hulled and halved fresh ripe or frozen unsweetened strawberries | 2 lb | 6 c (1½ qt) |
| Thawed white grape juice concentrate, undiluted | | ¾ c + 2 tbsp |
| Lemon juice | | 1 tbsp |
| Amaretto (almond-flavored) liqueur | | 2 tbsp |

Place strawberries, grape juice concentrate, and lemon juice in a food processor or blender. Blend until strawberries are smooth. Strain purée through a coarse mesh strainer. Pour mixture into freezer container of an ice cream freezer. Freeze according to manufacturer's instructions. When partially frozen, mix in amaretto. When frozen, serve immediately, or spoon into a covered airtight container and freeze.

Alternatively, to still-freeze glacé, pour ¼-inch layer of mixture into a nonreactive metal pan. Cover tightly and freeze until almost firm.

Break into small chunks with a heavy spoon. Process briefly in a food processor or blender, or beat in a mixing bowl until just slushy, beginning with mixer on low speed and increasing to medium as mixture softens.

Repeat freezing and beating 3 times at half-hour intervals. After beating third time, mix in amaretto. Serve or freeze until serving time. If glacé is frozen hard, place in refrigerator until slightly softened, or 15 to 20 minutes, before scooping. Scoop into 8 dessert dishes. Garnish with mint sprigs, if desired, and serve.

---

### NUTRITIONAL FACTS

Calories: 91 (5% from fat)  
Fat: .5 g (.1 g sat, .1 g mono, .2 g poly)  
Protein: .9 g and 4%

Carbohydrate: 20.7 g and 85%  
Alcohol: .9 g and 7%  
Fiber: 2.7 g  
Cholesterol: 0 mg

Iron: .5 mg  
Sodium: 3.1 mg  
Calcium: 19.3 mg  
Diabetic Exchanges: 1½ Fruits

# Strawberry Cheesecake Fat-Free Ice Cream

*Most Americans love both ice cream and cheesecake. Put them together, add juicy ripe strawberries, eliminate the fat and cholesterol, reduce the calories, and you've created this dessert. Americans are fond of ice cream any time of the year, and when the ice cream is as healthful as this version, you can feel free to indulge more often.*

YIELD: 5 c (1¼ qt) ice cream  SERVINGS: 10
SERVING SIZE: ½ c ice cream

| | WEIGHT | MEASURE |
|---|---|---|
| Hulled and halved fresh ripe or frozen unsweetened strawberries | 1 lb | 3 c (1½ pt) |
| Fat-free sweetened condensed milk | 14-oz can | |
| Block-style fat-free cream cheese, cubed | 1 lb | 2 c (1 pt) |
| Vanilla extract | | 1 tsp |
| Red food coloring | | 3 to 5 drops (optional) |

Place strawberries in a blender or food processor. Purée until smooth.

Combine strawberry purée, condensed milk, cream cheese, vanilla, and red food coloring (if using) in a medium mixing bowl. Beat with an electric mixer until well blended. Pour mixture into freezer container of an ice cream freezer. Freeze according to manufacturer's instructions. Serve immediately, or spoon into a covered airtight container and freeze.

Alternatively, to still-freeze ice cream, pour ¼-inch layer of mixture into a nonreactive metal pan. Cover tightly and freeze until almost firm.

Break into small chunks with a heavy spoon. Process briefly in a food processor or blender, or beat in a mixing bowl until just slushy, beginning with mixer on low speed and increasing to medium as mixture softens.

Repeat freezing and beating 3 times at half-hour intervals. Serve after final beating or freeze until serving time. If ice cream is frozen hard, place in refrigerator until slightly softened, or 15 to 20 minutes, before scooping. Scoop into 10 dessert dishes. Garnish with strawberry fans, if desired, and serve. To create strawberry fans, make several parallel thin slices with a small pointed knife from the berry's root end almost through the stem end. Fan out.

NUTRITIONAL FACTS

Calories: 168 (1% from fat)

Fat: .1 g (0 g sat, 0 g mono, 0 g poly)

Protein: 10.6 g and 25%

Carbohydrate: 30.9 g and 74%

Fiber: 1 g

Cholesterol: 6 mg

Iron: .4 mg

Sodium: 262.5 mg

Calcium: 262.1 mg

Diabetic Exchanges: ½

Other Carbohydrate; ½

Fruit; 1 Skim Milk

# Strawberry Swirled Vanilla Frozen Yogurt Pie on Crispy Rice Crust

*This crunchy-crusted pie is filled with smooth and creamy vanilla low-fat strawberry swirl frozen yogurt and drizzled with bright red strawberry sauce. It is what "good-lookin' healthy cookin'" is all about. While it may sound complicated, it is easy to make. Add variety to your menu by replacing the vanilla-strawberry frozen yogurt with another flavor, and topping with a complementary sugar-free and low-fat sauce.*

YIELD: 9-inch pie                    SERVINGS: 8
SERVING SIZE: 1 wedge (one-eighth pie)

|  | WEIGHT | MEASURE |
|---|---|---|
| Vanilla low-fat frozen strawberry swirl yogurt, softened | 27 oz | 4 c (1 qt) |
| Crispy Rice Marshmallow Crust (page 169) |  | 1 recipe |
| Fruit Juice–Sweetened Strawberry Sauce (page 220), |  | 1 recipe |
| or fat-free strawberry ice cream topping |  | 1½ c + 3 tbsp |

Spoon softened frozen yogurt into 9-inch Crispy Rice Marshmallow Crust. Smooth with a spatula. Freeze until set.

Cut into 8 wedges. Ladle 3⅓ tablespoons Fruit Juice–Sweetened Strawberry Sauce over each piece. Garnish with fresh mint sprigs and/or strawberry fans (page 200), if desired, and serve. Wedges of this pie also look spectacular presented on plates decorated with strawberry sauce piped from a squeeze bottle into swirls or geometric designs.

---

### NUTRITIONAL FACTS

Calories: 238 (6% from fat)
Fat: 1.6 g (.9 g sat, .4 g mono, .1 g poly)
Protein: 5.5 g and 9%

Carbohydrate: 52.5 g and 85%
Fiber: .8 g
Cholesterol: 5.1 mg
Iron: 1.1 mg
Sodium: 187.6 mg

Calcium: 175.5 mg
Diabetic Exchanges: ½ Starch; 2 Other Carbohydrates; ½ Fruit; ½ Low-Fat Milk

---

# Smoothies, Shakes, Fruit Drinks, and Teas

Banana-Strawberry Smoothie with Soy Milk

Blended Watermelon Cooler Flavored with Mint

East Indian–Style Tea with Spices (Chai)

Fresh-Squeezed Lemonade Sweetened with Honey

Mango and Strawberry Yogurt Smoothie

Naturally Sweetened Banana Shake

Peaches and Just-Like-Cream Smoothie

Tropical Fruit and Green Tea Julep

# Banana-Strawberry Smoothie with Soy Milk

*With its smooth, creamy texture and mild sweetness, soy milk can be used in almost any way that cow's milk is used. It might be served chilled as a refreshing beverage, poured over both cold and hot breakfast cereals, mixed into puddings, creamy soups, macaroni and cheese, pancakes, waffles or French toast, or blended with fruit for a protein-, vitamin-, and mineral-rich smoothie. Soy milk is most commonly aseptically packaged but is also sold refrigerated. To maximize the taste and nutritional value yet minimize the calories and fat in this creamy pink smoothie, lite vanilla soy milk is blended with bananas, strawberries, and fruit juice concentrate.*

YIELD: 4½ c (1⅛ qt)   SERVINGS: 6
SERVING SIZE: ¾ c

|  | WEIGHT | MEASURE |
|---|---|---|
| Ripe banana, peeled and sliced | 6 oz | 1 medium |
| Fresh ripe and hulled strawberries, or frozen unsweetened strawberries | 6 oz | 1 c |
| Lite vanilla soy milk |  | 2 c (1 pt) |
| Thawed orange juice concentrate, undiluted |  | ¼ c |
| Thawed white grape juice concentrate, undiluted |  | ¼ c |
| Crushed or cracked ice |  | ½ c |

Combine banana, strawberries, soy milk, juice concentrates, and ice in a blender or food processor. Blend until smooth. Pour into 6 chilled stemmed glasses. Garnish with strawberry fans (page 200), if desired, and serve.

---

### NUTRITIONAL FACTS

Calories: 113 (7% from fat)
Fat: .9 g (.2 g sat, .2 g mono, .4 g poly)
Protein: 3.7 g and 12%

Carbohydrate: 24 g and 81%
Fiber: 2.2 g
Cholesterol: 0 mg
Iron: 1 mg

Sodium: 32.9 mg
Calcium: 96.8 mg
Diabetic Exchanges: 1 Fruit; ½ Skim Milk

# Blended Watermelon Cooler Flavored with Mint

*When blessed with an abundance of ripe, sweet, juicy watermelon, blend it with fruit juice concentrate, a splash of lime juice, and some fresh mint to make this refreshing, cooling beverage. Use the familiar red-fleshed watermelon or the orange- or yellow-fleshed variety—there will be little difference in taste between the three.*

YIELD: 2 c (1 pt)  SERVINGS: 2
SERVING SIZE: 1 c

|  | WEIGHT | MEASURE |
|---|---|---|
| Seedless watermelon cubes, chilled | 17 oz | 3 c (1½ pt) |
| Thawed white grape juice concentrate, undiluted |  | 3 tbsp |
| Fresh lime juice |  | 1½ tbsp |
| Fresh mint leaves |  | 3 |

Combine watermelon, grape juice concentrate, lime juice, and mint leaves in a blender or food processor. Blend until smooth. Pour into 2 tall chilled glasses. Garnish with mint sprigs, if desired, and serve.

---

### NUTRITIONAL FACTS

Calories: 129 (7% from fat)

Fat: 1.1g (.1 g sat, .3 g mono, .4 g poly)

Protein: 1.7 g and 5%

Carbohydrate: 30.3 g and 88%

Fiber: 1.3 g

Cholesterol: 0 mg

Iron: .5 mg

Sodium: 6.8 mg

Calcium: 23.8 mg

Diabetic Exchanges: 2 Fruits

# East Indian–Style Tea with Spices (Chai)

*My first experience with chai was on a visit to India. Today, my East Indian–born husband, Tarun, makes this spicy milk tea in our home on a daily basis. This recipe is his version of the fragrant hot beverage. As in India, a soothing cup can be enjoyed any time of the day.*

YIELD: 1½ c                                      SERVINGS: 2
SERVING SIZE: ¾ c

|  | WEIGHT | MEASURE |
|---|---|---|
| Cold water, filtered or tap (not distilled) |  | 1 c |
| Low-fat milk |  | ½ c |
| Green or white cardamom pods, lightly crushed |  | 2 |
| 1-inch-piece cinnamon stick, broken in half |  | 1 |
| 1⅛-inch-thick slice fresh ginger |  | 1 |
| Assam or orange pekoe tea bags, |  | 2 |
|    or loose Assam or orange pekoe tea |  | 2 heaping tsp |

Combine water and milk in a small saucepan. Heat to a boil, then remove from heat. Add cardamom, cinnamon, and ginger, and mix. Cover and set to infuse spices, at least 10 minutes.

    Add tea bags or tea to pan. Heat to boiling, then reduce heat to low and simmer, covered, 5 minutes. Preheat 2 cups by filling with boiling or very hot water, then draining. Strain tea into cups and serve immediately. Offer honey or another sweetener, if desired. (Note: This will not be included in the nutrition analysis.)

---

### NUTRITIONAL FACTS

Calories: 28 (20% from fat)

Fat: .6 g (.4 g sat, .1 g mono, 0 g poly)

Protein: 2.3 g and 33%

Carbohydrate: 3.3 g and 47%

Fiber: 0 g

Cholesterol: 3.8 mg

Iron: 0 mg

Sodium: 32.5 mg

Calcium: 67.5 mg

Diabetic Exchanges: Free Food

# Fresh-Squeezed Lemonade Sweetened with Honey

*There's nothing like a tall glass of fresh-squeezed lemonade on the rocks when the temperature skyrockets. This honey-sweetened version is prepared with sparkling mineral water but can be made with tap water, too. On special occasions, insert a colorful straw through a thin slice of lemon and float it on top, or offer the tangy beverage topped with a knotted thin strip of bright yellow lemon peel and a sprig of mint. Lemon slices or wedges frozen on swizzle sticks and dredged in granulated sugar or colored candy sprinkles or brushed with fruit spread make attractive lemonade garnishes, too.*

YIELD: 4 c (1 qt)                    SERVINGS: 4
SERVING SIZE: 1 c

|  | WEIGHT | MEASURE |
| --- | --- | --- |
| Honey |  | ¼ c |
| Boiling water |  | ¼ c |
| Fresh lemon juice |  | ½ c (3 lemons) |
| Sparkling mineral or tap water |  | 3 c (1½ pt) |

Combine honey and boiling water in a heat-resistant pitcher or bowl. Stir until dissolved. Add lemon juice and water. Stir until blended.

Pour lemonade into 4 tall chilled glasses filled with ice. Decorate with a lemon garnish, if desired, and serve.

### LEMON GARNISHES

Lemon Wedges Dredged in Minced Mint: Cut a thin slice from each end of a lemon with a small, sharp, pointed knife to enhance its appearance. Cut into quarters. Remove any seeds. Dip top edge or one side of each lemon wedge in finely minced mint for added color.

Lemon Knots: Cut a thin slice from each end of a lemon with a small, sharp, pointed knife. Stand lemon on end. Cut peel from top to bottom in long thin strips with knife tip. Tie each strip in a knot, being careful not to break it. Use peeled fruit to make fresh juice.

Floating Lemon Slices: Float a thin slice of lemon on top of lemonade and insert a colorful straw through its center.

Candy-Coated Frozen Lemon Slices: Freeze lemon slices on swizzle sticks. Dredge both sides in granulated sugar or colored candy sprinkles or brush with a fruit spread, such as 100%-fruit strawberry spread, and place on drinks.

---

### NUTRITIONAL FACTS

| | | |
|---|---|---|
| Calories: 72 (0% from fat) | Fiber: .2 g | Calcium: 7 mg |
| Fat: 0 g | Cholesterol: 0 mg | Diabetic Exchanges: 1 |
| Protein: .2 g and 1% | Iron: .1 mg |     Other Carbohydrate; ½ |
| Carbohydrate: 20.1 g and 99% | Sodium: 8.5 mg |     Fruit |

---

# Mango and Strawberry Yogurt Smoothie

*The mango is ready for this smoothie when it smells good. This beta-carotene-rich golden fruit should never be stored in the refrigerator. As for the strawberries, they are picked when ripe, so purchase no more than a day or two before you're ready to use them. Strawberries contain a lot of vitamin C, and one-half cup of the berries provides more fiber than a slice of whole wheat bread. These two fruits are blended with fat-free plain yogurt, an excellent source of protein and calcium and a good source of riboflavin, phosphorous, and vitamin $B_{12}$, making this creamy beverage a nutritional powerhouse.*

YIELD: 3 c (1½ pt)                                        SERVINGS: 4
SERVING SIZE: ¾ c

| | WEIGHT | MEASURE |
|---|---|---|
| Ripe mango, peeled, pitted, and cubed | 1 lb as purchased | 1 large |
| Fresh ripe strawberries, hulled, or unsweetened frozen strawberries | 4 oz | ¾ c |
| Fat-free plain yogurt | 4 oz | ½ c |
| Thawed white grape juice concentrate, undiluted | | ¼ c |
| Crushed or cracked ice | | 1 c |

Combine mango, strawberries, yogurt, grape juice concentrate, and ice in a blender or food processor. Process until smooth. Pour into 4 chilled stemmed glasses. Garnish with strawberry fans (page 200) or colorful straws, if desired, and serve.

---

### NUTRITIONAL FACTS

Calories: 86 (3% from fat)
Fat: .3 g (.1 g sat, .1 g mono, .1 g poly)
Protein: 1.5 g and 6%

Carbohydrate: 20.8 g and 90%
Fiber: 1.7 g
Cholesterol: .3 mg
Iron: .3 mg

Sodium: 14.5 mg
Calcium: 42.5 mg
Diabetic Exchanges: 1½ Fruits

---

# Naturally Sweetened Banana Shake

*To create this rich-tasting, low-fat, and sugar-free shake, creamy ripe bananas are blended with fat-free half-and-half, apple juice concentrate, and ice. Besides being the least expensive and most popular fruit in the market, bananas rate tops in nutritional value. They are good sources of vitamin $B_6$, potassium, and fiber; low in sodium and fat; and cholesterol-free. And according to a University of California study, the risk of stroke can be* *reduced by as much as 40 percent by simply eating one banana a day. As for fat-free half-and-half, it contains only 10 calories and less than 2 grams of fat per tablespoon, yet looks and tastes like the full-fat kind. It is made of mostly fat-free milk (with carrageenan added for texture). The third ingredient on the list, apple juice concentrate, provides fruity sugar-free sweetness, and finally, ice is added to chill the creamy nutritious beverage and mellow out its flavor. For a finishing touch, toasted flaked sweetened coconut is sprinkled on top.*

YIELD: 2 c (1 pt)                                              SERVINGS: 4
SERVING SIZE: ½ c

|  | WEIGHT | MEASURE |
|---|---|---|
| Ripe bananas, peeled and sliced | 12 oz as purchased | 2 medium |
| Fat-free half-and-half |  | ¼ c |
| Thawed apple juice concentrate, undiluted |  | ¼ c |
| Crushed or cracked ice |  | 1 c |
| Flaked sweetened coconut, toasted without oil |  | 4 tsp |

Combine all ingredients through ice in a blender or food processor. Blend until smooth. Pour into 4 chilled, stemmed glasses. Sprinkle each with 1 teaspoon toasted coconut and serve. (Toast coconut by cooking over medium heat in a dry nonstick skillet, stirring constantly until golden brown.)

---

NUTRITIONAL FACTS

Calories: 119 (7% from fat)
Fat: 1 g (.6 g sat, .1 g mono, .1 g poly)
Protein: 1.5 g and 5%

Carbohydrate: 28 g and 88%
Fiber: 2.2 g
Cholesterol: 0 mg
Iron: .4 mg

Sodium: 20.7 mg
Calcium: 8.2 mg
Diabetic Exchanges: 2 Fruits

# Peaches and Just-Like-Cream Smoothie

*Juicy golden peach slices are blended with fat-free half-and-half and a tad of fruit juice concentrate to make this sweet and creamy sugar-free smoothie. If you've ever wondered why the peaches at farmers' markets and roadside stands have a fuzzy beard on their skin while the ones sold at supermarkets don't, it's because commercially grown peaches are mechanically brushed after harvest to remove their fuzz.*

YIELD: 2 c (1 pt)                    SERVINGS: 4
SERVING SIZE: ½ c

| | WEIGHT | MEASURE |
|---|---|---|
| Ripe peach, peeled, pitted, and sliced | 9 oz as purchased | 1 large |
| Fat-free half-and-half | | ¼ c + 2 tbsp |
| Thawed white grape juice concentrate, undiluted | | ¼ c |
| Crushed or cracked ice | | 1 c |

To peel the peach, blanch it in boiling water for 20 to 60 seconds and then place in ice water or under cold running water until completely cooled. The skin should slip off easily. Or use 7½ ounces (1¼ cups) frozen unsweetened peach slices, if desired.

Combine peach slices, half-and-half, grape juice concentrate, and ice in a blender or food processor. Process until smooth. Pour into 4 chilled, stemmed glasses. Garnish with peeled peach slices threaded on small skewers, if desired, and serve.

| NUTRITIONAL FACTS | | |
|---|---|---|
| Calories: 68 (1% from fat) | Carbohydrate: 15.6 g and 92% | Sodium: 19.7 mg |
| Fat: .1 g | | Calcium: 4.8 mg |
| Protein: 1.2 g and 7% | Fiber: 1 g | Diabetic Exchanges: 1 Fruit |
| | Cholesterol: 0 mg | |
| | Iron: .1 mg | |

# Tropical Fruit and Green Tea Julep

*Ever since tea took on a healthful aura, commercial iced tea concoctions have abounded in the marketplace. Many have lots of added sugar, and that means lots of empty calories. There's a simple solution: Make your own.*

*To brew tea, place 1 teaspoon of loose tea or one tea bag per ¾ cup water in a warmed teapot; pour the appropriate amount of just-boiled water over; cover with the teapot lid and infuse for 3 to 5 minutes. Remove the loose tea leaves or tea bag from the water when brewing is complete. Do not use color as an indicator of brewing time. Tea leaves release color before flavor, and the desired color of properly brewed tea varies among types.*

YIELD: 3 c (1½ pt)　　　　　　　　　　　　　　　　SERVINGS: 3
SERVING SIZE: 1 c

|  | WEIGHT | MEASURE |
|---|---|---|
| Ripe papaya, peeled, seeded, and cut into 1-inch cubes | 1 lb as purchased | 1 medium (1 c cubes) |
| Fresh ripe or canned-in-juice and drained 1-inch pineapple cubes | 6 oz | 1 c |
| Brewed green tea, chilled |  | 1 c |
| Thawed white grape juice concentrate, undiluted |  | 2 tbsp |

Combine all ingredients in a blender or food processor. Blend until smooth. Pour over ice in tall glasses and serve.

---

### NUTRITIONAL FACTS

| | | |
|---|---|---|
| Calories: 114 (2% from fat) | Carbohydrate: 29.1 g and 94% | Sodium: 8.3 mg |
| Fat: .3 g (.1 g sat, .1 g mono, .1 g poly) | Fiber: 3.2 g | Calcium: 47.4 mg |
| Protein: 1.2 g and 4% | Cholesterol: 0 mg | Diabetic Exchanges: 2 Fruits |
| | Iron: .4 mg | |

# Frostings, Sauces, Dips, and Toppings

Apple-Flavored Caramel Glaze with a Splash of Brandy

Cocoa Mocha Frosting

Creamy Vanilla Custard Sauce Spiked with Amaretto

Dairy-Fresh Sour Cream Frosting

Fresh Kiwi Coulis

Fresh Mango Coulis

Fruit Juice–Sweetened Strawberry Sauce

Lemon Powdered Sugar Frosting with Finely Grated Zest

Lemon Sauce Dancing with Lemon, Lime, and Orange Zests

Orange Powdered Sugar Frosting with Finely Grated Zest

Pumpkin Pie Cheesecake Dip

Quick-and-Easy Chocolate Icing

Raspberry Sauce Sweetened with Fruit Juice

Summer-Fresh Three Berry Sauce

Whipped Light Cream Cheese Frosting

# Apple-Flavored Caramel Glaze with a Splash of Brandy

*Caramel sauce is typically prepared from "burnt" sugar that has been thinned with a mixture of butter, cream, water, or other liquid. In this recipe, granulated sugar is mixed and cooked with apple juice and a splash of brandy. The result is a clear, mahogany-colored caramel sauce with a light apple flavor.*

YIELD: 1½ c glaze
SERVING SIZE: about 2½ tbsp glaze

SERVINGS: 10

|  | WEIGHT | MEASURE |
|---|---|---|
| Granulated sugar | 12 oz | 1⅔ c |
| Thawed apple juice concentrate, undiluted |  | ½ c + 2 tbsp |
| Water |  | ½ c |
| Brandy |  | 3 tbsp |

Combine all ingredients in a medium saucepan. Heat to boiling, stirring until sugar is dissolved. Cover and cook until steam washes down sides of pan, or about 3 minutes.

Uncover and reduce heat to simmer. Cook, without stirring, until sauce reaches 220 degrees F on a candy thermometer. Remove from heat. If sauce becomes too thick, heat and thin to desired consistency with water.

Serve warm over desserts such as Sweet Potato Cheesecake Drizzled with Apple-Flavored Caramel Glaze (page 164).

---

NUTRITIONAL FACTS

Calories: 159 (0% from fat)
Fat: .1 g
Protein: .1 g and 0%

Carbohydrate: 39.8 g and 97%
Alcohol: .6 g and 2%
Fiber: .1 g
Cholesterol: 0 mg
Iron: .2 mg

Sodium: 4.3 mg
Calcium: 3.4 mg
Diabetic Exchanges: 2
Other Carbohydrates; ½ Fruit

---

# Cocoa Mocha Frosting

*Mocha (moh-kuh) refers to the flavor that results from combining coffee and chocolate. In this frosting, double-strength decaffeinated coffee is blended with cocoa powder, powdered sugar, and malted milk powder.*

YIELD: ¾ c frosting      SERVINGS: 24
SERVING SIZE: ½ tbsp frosting

| | WEIGHT | MEASURE |
|---|---|---|
| Sifted powdered sugar | 5 oz | 1¼ c |
| Malted-milk powder | | 2 tbsp |
| Unsweetened cocoa powder | | 2 tbsp |
| Double-strength decaffeinated coffee, hot | | 2 tbsp |

Combine all ingredients in a small bowl. Whisk until smooth and of spreading consistency. Spread evenly over cookies, cakes, and bars such as Coconut-Flavored Chocolate Brownie Bars (page 97) and serve.

---

### NUTRITIONAL FACTS

Calories: 31 (6% from fat)
Fat: .2 g (.1 g sat, .1 g mono, 0 g poly)
Protein: .3 g and 3%

Carbohydrate: 7.5 g and 91%
Fiber: .2 g
Cholesterol: .4 mg
Iron: .1 mg

Sodium: 8.8 mg
Calcium: 5.9 mg
Diabetic Exchanges: ½ Other Carbohydrate

---

# Creamy Vanilla Custard Sauce Spiked with Amaretto

*While this custard sauce calls for about 20 minutes of cooking and stirring, it's worth it. Dolloped on warm aromatic gingerbread cake or layered with sliced fresh fruit, this smooth and creamy vanilla-flavored sauce* with a hint of almond will remind you of eating soft vanilla ice cream. To reduce the fat and calories, and to obtain a rich vanilla flavor, whole milk is replaced with low-fat milk in which a vanilla bean is steeped. A splash of almond-flavored liqueur finishes it with a light, nutty essence.

YIELD: 2 c (1 pt) sauce        SERVINGS: 4
SERVING SIZE: ½ c sauce

| | WEIGHT | MEASURE |
| --- | --- | --- |
| Low-fat milk | | 2 c (1 pt) |
| Vanilla bean split lengthwise, or 1 tsp vanilla extract | | 3- to 4-inch piece |
| Granulated sugar | 4 oz | ½ c |
| Large eggs | 4 oz | 2 |
| Large egg whites | 2½ oz | 2 |
| Amaretto (almond-flavored liqueur) | | 2 tsp |

Combine milk and vanilla bean in a medium saucepan. Heat to a boil, stirring constantly. Remove from heat. Cover and set to steep 30 minutes. If using vanilla extract, heat milk only. Vanilla extract will be added at end of cooking.

Meanwhile, combine sugar, eggs, and egg whites in a small bowl. Beat until well mixed.

Temper egg mixture by gradually beating about ⅓ of the warm milk into it. Beating, pour egg-milk mixture into remaining milk.

Cook sauce mixture over medium-low heat, stirring constantly until mixture thickens to consistency of thin pudding, or about 20 minutes. Do not boil or sauce will curdle. Remove from heat. Stir until slightly cooled. Strain sauce through a fine mesh strainer into a bowl. Rinse vanilla bean, dry, and reserve for another use.

Stir in amaretto and vanilla extract, if using. Cover sauce and refrigerate until chilled. Layer with Summer Fruit Layered with Vanilla Amaretto Custard Sauce (page 31) or spoon over moist and dense homestyle cakes such as Gingerbread Cake Laced with Fresh Ginger (page 68) and serve.

```
┌─────────────────────────────────────────────────────────────┐
│                    NUTRITIONAL FACTS                          │
│                                                               │
│  Calories: 215 (16% from    Carbohydrate: 35.7 g and   Sodium: 120.9 mg          │
│     fat)                       66%                     Calcium: 163.6 mg          │
│  Fat: 3.8 g (1.6 g sat, 1.3 g   Alcohol: .6 g and 2%   Diabetic Exchanges: 2      │
│     mono, .4 g poly)         Fiber: 0 g                  Other Carbohydrates;     │
│  Protein: 8.9 g and 16%      Cholesterol: 111.1 mg       1 Lean Meat; ½ Skim      │
│                              Iron: .4 mg                 Milk                     │
└─────────────────────────────────────────────────────────────┘
```

# Dairy-Fresh Sour Cream Frosting

*The fat-free sour cream called for in this recipe obtains its light tang from fat-free milk cultured with lactic acid bacteria. To make your own fat-free sour cream, simply whip a small amount of commercial fat-free sour cream with fat-free milk until the mixture is quite runny. Then refrigerate to cure for a day or two or until it thickens.*

YIELD: ⅝ c frosting                                      SERVINGS: 9
SERVING SIZE: 3⅓ tsp frosting

|  | WEIGHT | MEASURE |
|---|---|---|
| Fat-free sour cream | 4 oz | ½ c |
| Sifted powdered sugar | 3 oz | ¾ c |

Combine sour cream and powdered sugar in a small bowl. Whisk until well blended. Spread over cookies and cakes such as Homestyle Banana Cake Enriched with Sour Cream (page 73) and serve.

```
┌─────────────────────────────────────────────────────────────┐
│                    NUTRITIONAL FACTS                          │
│                                                               │
│  Calories: 45 (0% from fat)   Fiber: 0 g        Calcium: .1 mg│
│  Fat: 0 g                     Cholesterol: 0 mg Diabetic Exchanges: │
│  Protein: .9 g and 8%         Iron: 0 mg            ½ Other Carbohydrate │
│  Carbohydrate: 10.7 g and     Sodium: 9 mg        │
│     92%                                                       │
└─────────────────────────────────────────────────────────────┘
```

# Fresh Kiwi Coulis

*For an easy but elegant, light and refreshing, sugar-free and low-fat dessert with lots of nutrients and fiber, drizzle this fruit juice–sweetened kiwi purée on a large dinner plate and decorate with a medley of brightly colored slices of fresh, ripe, sweet fruit and berries. Kiwi coulis is best served the day it is made, as its color fades over time.*

YIELD: 1¼ c coulis and 2½ c fruit          SERVINGS: 5
SERVING SIZE: ¼ c coulis and ½ c fruit

|  | WEIGHT | MEASURE |
|---|---|---|
| Kiwis, divided | 1½ lb as purchased | 8 medium |
| Thawed apple juice concentrate, undiluted |  | 2 tbsp |
| Thawed white grape juice concentrate, undiluted |  | 2 tbsp |
| Lime juice |  | 2 tsp |
| Fresh ripe hulled and sliced strawberries | 6 oz | 1 c |
| Fresh ripe blueberries | 5 oz | 1 c |

Peel and coarsely chop 5 kiwis. Combine chopped kiwis, juice concentrates, and lime juice in a blender or food processor. Blend only until smooth. Be careful not to overprocess and mash kiwis' seeds, as sauce will turn brown.

Peel and slice remaining 3 kiwis ¼ inch thick. Ladle kiwi coulis on 5 dessert plates. Arrange sliced kiwis and strawberries and blueberries attractively on top and serve.

For a stylish dessert, ladle kiwi coulis with Fresh Mango Coulis (below) in a decorative pattern on a large white plate. Top with sliced kiwis and 3 small scoops of strawberry sorbet such as Strawberry Amaretto Glacé (page 198). Garnish with sliced strawberries and blueberries, if desired.

---

### NUTRITIONAL FACTS

| | | |
|---|---|---|
| Calories: 132 (5% from fat) | Carbohydrate: 32.4 g and 89% | Sodium: 10.8 mg |
| Fat: .9 g (.1 g sat, .1 g mono, .5 g poly) | Fiber: 6.2 g | Calcium: 44.1 mg |
| Protein: 1.8 g and 5% | Cholesterol: 0 mg | Diabetic Exchanges: 2 Fruits |
| | Iron: .8 mg | |

---

# Fresh Mango Coulis

*The term* coulis *is used to describe a variety of dishes including both fruit and vegetable sauces.* The New Food Lover's Companion *defines it as a general term for a thick purée or sauce. So both this fresh mango sauce as well as a cooked tomato sauce would meet the criteria.*

YIELD: 1 c coulis                                                          SERVINGS: 4
SERVING SIZE: ¼ c coulis

| | WEIGHT | MEASURE |
|---|---|---|
| Ripe mango, peeled, pitted, and cubed | 1 lb as purchased | 1 medium |
| Thawed white grape juice concentrate, undiluted | | 2 tbsp |
| Lime juice | | 2 tsp |

Combine all ingredients in a blender or food processor. Blend until smooth. Spoon over sliced fresh fruit or whole grain pancakes or French toast and serve immediately, or chill up to 3 days.

For an elegant dessert, ladle mango coulis with Fresh Kiwi Coulis (page 218) in a decorative pattern on a large plate. Top with 3 small scoops of strawberry sorbet such as Strawberry Amaretto Glacé (page 198) and garnish with sliced strawberries and blueberries, if desired. It can also be drizzled over sliced bananas and then sprinkled with toasted flaked sweetened coconut.

---

### NUTRITIONAL FACTS

Calories: 91 (3% from fat)  
Fat: .3 g (.1 g sat, .1 g mono, .1 g poly)  
Protein: .7 g and 3%  

Carbohydrate: 23.5 g and 94%  
Fiber: 2.1 g  
Cholesterol: 0 mg  
Iron: .2 mg  

Sodium: 2.9 mg  
Calcium: 12.7 mg  
Diabetic Exchanges: 1½ Fruits  

---

# Fruit Juice–Sweetened Strawberry Sauce

*In addition to being one of American's favorite fruits, strawberries are a well-known symbol of love and romance. So when love is in the air, offer this strawberry sauce over a slice of angel food cake or a scoop of vanilla low-fat ice cream. For best flavor and appearance, don't wash or hull the berries before refrigerating. Their caps prevent water from entering and breaking down their interiors.*

YIELD: 1¾ c sauce  
SERVING SIZE: 3 tbsp sauce  

SERVINGS: 9

|  | WEIGHT | MEASURE |
|---|---|---|
| Hulled fresh ripe strawberries or unsweetened frozen strawberries | 9 oz | 1⅔ c |
| Peeled very ripe banana slices | 3 oz | ½ c |
| Thawed white grape juice concentrate, undiluted |  | 2 tbsp |

Combine all ingredients in a blender or food processor. Purée until smooth. Spoon over frozen desserts such as Strawberry Swirled Vanilla Frozen Yogurt Pie on Crispy Rice Crust (page 201) and serve.

---

### NUTRITIONAL FACTS

Calories: 26 (4% from fat)

Fat: .1 g (0 g sat, 0 g mono, 0 g poly)

Protein: .2 g and 3%

Carbohydrate: 6.4 g and 92%

Fiber: .6 g

Cholesterol: 0 mg

Iron: .3 mg

Sodium: .9 mg

Calcium: 18.2 mg

Diabetic Exchanges: ½ Fruit

---

# Lemon Powdered Sugar Frosting with Finely Grated Zest

*What do Dried Plum Cake Flavored with Aromatic Spices (page 65), Carrot Raisin Cookies Topped with Lemon Frosting (page 92), and Soft Molasses Sour Cream Cookies (page 105) have in common? This lemon-flavored powdered sugar icing is delicious on all three.*

YIELD: ½ c frosting

SERVINGS: 48

SERVING SIZE: ½ tsp frosting

| | WEIGHT | MEASURE |
|---|---|---|
| Sifted powdered sugar | 6 oz | 1½ c |
| Fresh lemon juice | | 3 tbsp |
| Finely grated lemon zest | | ⅛ tsp |

Combine all ingredients in a small bowl. Beat until smooth and of spreading consistency. Serve spread over cakes, cookies, and bars.

## VARIATION

Maple Powdered Sugar Frosting: Substitute 3 tablespoons maple syrup for lemon juice and lemon zest. Spread on cakes such as Aromatic Applesauce Spice Cake Studded with Raisins (page 60), bars, and cookies such as Applesauce Spice Cookies Dotted with Raisins (page 90) and serve.

---

### NUTRITIONAL FACTS

Calories: 14 (0% from fat)   Fiber: 0 g   Calcium: .1 mg

Fat: 0 g   Cholesterol: 0 mg   Diabetic Exchanges: Free

Protein: 0 g and 0%   Iron: 0 mg   Food

Carbohydrate: 3.6 g and   Sodium: .1 mg
  100%

---

# Lemon Sauce Dancing with Lemon, Lime, and Orange Zests

*Traditionally, lemon sauce was enriched with butter. There's no need when the sauce is made from a mixture of freshly squeezed lemon, lime, and orange juices and their finely grated zests. To obtain the maximum juice from citrus fruits, set them at room temperature or slightly warm the fruits in the microwave, and then roll them, while pressing at the same time, on a flat work surface.*

YIELD: 2½ c (1¼ pt) sauce          SERVINGS: 20
SERVING SIZE: 2 tbsp sauce

| | WEIGHT | MEASURE |
|---|---|---|
| Cornstarch | | ¼ c |
| Water, divided | 12 oz | 1⅔ c |
| Finely grated lemon zest | | 1 tsp |
| Finely grated lime zest | | 1 tsp |
| Finely grated orange zest | | 1 tsp |
| Fresh lemon juice | | ¼ c |
| Fresh lime juice | | 3 tbsp |
| Fresh orange juice | | 2 tbsp |
| Granulated sugar | | 1¾ c |
| Yellow food coloring | | 2 drops (optional) |

Combine cornstarch and ¼ cup water in a small bowl. Mix until smooth. Set aside.

Prepare lemon, lime, and orange zests. Set aside. Squeeze lemon, lime, and orange juices.

Combine juices, remaining 1½ cups water, and sugar in a medium saucepan. Heat to boiling, stirring constantly for about 2 minutes.

Whisk cornstarch mixture into sauce, beating constantly until thick and smooth, or about 10 seconds. Remove from heat.

Stir in zests and food coloring, if using. Ladle warm, at room temperature, or chilled over cakes such as Gingerbread Cake Laced with Fresh Ginger (page 68) or creamy frozen desserts such as vanilla fat-free frozen yogurt and serve.

---

### NUTRITIONAL FACTS

Calories: 75 (0% from fat)
Fat: 0 g
Protein: 0 g and 0%
Carbohydrate: 19.4 g and 100%

Fiber: .1 g
Cholesterol: 0 mg
Iron: 0 mg
Sodium: 1.1 mg;

Calcium: 1.6 mg
Diabetic Exchanges:
1½ Other Carbohydrates

# Orange Powdered Sugar Frosting with Finely Grated Zest

*This frosting, like most, should only be applied to a completely cooled cake. If not, the cake will stick to the spreader and the icing will become loose and runny.*

YIELD: ⅝ c frosting

SERVINGS: 60

SERVING SIZE: ½ tsp frosting

| | WEIGHT | MEASURE |
|---|---|---|
| Sifted powdered sugar | 6 oz | 1½ c |
| Thawed orange juice concentrate, undiluted | | 1½ tbsp |
| Water | | 1 tbsp |
| Finely grated orange zest | | 1½ tsp |

Combine all ingredients in a small bowl. Beat until smooth and of spreading consistency. Spread on cakes such as Moist Bran Cake Sprinkled with Dried Cranberries (page 77), and bars and cookies such as Golden Pumpkin Cookies Spiked with Date Bits (page 99) and serve.

---

### NUTRITIONAL FACTS

Calories: 12 (0% from fat)
Fat: 0 g
Protein: 0 g and 0%
Carbohydrate: 3 g and 99%

Fiber: 0 g
Cholesterol: 0 mg
Iron: 0 mg
Sodium: .1 mg

Calcium: .3 mg
Diabetic Exchanges: Free Food

# Pumpkin Pie Cheesecake Dip

*This dip has all the taste of pumpkin pie, with the smooth and creamy texture of cream cheese. Yet it contains no fat and only 26 calories per tablespoon. To achieve its rich, appealing taste, pumpkin is blended with powdered sugar, fat-free cream cheese, pumpkin pie spices, and crystallized ginger.*

YIELD: 2⅛ c dip                    SERVINGS: 34
SERVING SIZE: 1 tbsp dip

| | WEIGHT | MEASURE |
|---|---|---|
| Block-style fat-free cream cheese, softened | 6 oz | ¾ c |
| Sifted powdered sugar | 6 oz | 1½ c |
| Canned pumpkin | 8 oz | scant 1 c |
| Minced crystallized ginger | | ½ tbsp |
| Ground cinnamon | | ½ tsp |
| Ground ginger | | ¼ tsp |
| Ground allspice | | ⅛ tsp |
| Ground cloves | | pinch |

Place cream cheese in a medium mixing bowl. Beat with an electric mixer until smooth and creamy. Gradually add sugar, beating until well mixed.

Add pumpkin, crystallized ginger, cinnamon, ground ginger, allspice, and cloves. Mix until well blended.

Serve fondu-style with sliced fruit such as crisp Asian pear or apple slices or cubes of low-fat cake such as angel food cake or Gingerbread Cake Laced with Fresh Ginger (page 68). It can also be offered as an alternative to cream cheese, butter, margarine, jam, or jelly with assorted breads. Pipe in decorative individual servings, if desired. Store refrigerated.

---

### NUTRITIONAL FACTS

| | | |
|---|---|---|
| Calories: 26 (1% from fat) | Fiber: .1 g | Calcium: 1.6 mg |
| Fat: 0 g | Cholesterol: .9 mg | Diabetic Exchanges: |
| Protein: .8 g and 12% | Iron: .1 mg | ½ Other Carbohydrate |
| Carbohydrate: 5.6 g and 88% | Sodium: 30.2 mg | |

# Quick-and-Easy Chocolate Icing

*The sweetening agent in this frosting is powdered sugar, also known as confectioners' sugar. It is granulated sugar that has been ground into a fine powder. To prevent caking, a small amount (about 3 percent) of cornstarch is added. Powdered sugar is a useful sweetening agent in uncooked frostings because it readily dissolves.*

YIELD: ¾ c frosting
SERVING SIZE: ½ tbsp frosting

SERVINGS: 24

| | WEIGHT | MEASURE |
|---|---|---|
| Sifted powdered sugar | 5 oz | 1¼ c |
| Unsweetened cocoa powder | 1 oz | ¼ c |
| Fat-free milk | | 3 tbsp |
| Vanilla extract | | ½ tsp |

Combine all ingredients in a small bowl. Beat until smooth and of spreading consistency. For a thinner consistency, add more milk. (Note: This will not be included in nutrition analysis.) Spread on cakes, cookies, and bars such as Chocolate Brownies Just Like Mom's (page 94) and serve.

---

### NUTRITIONAL FACTS

Calories: 27 (5% from fat)
Fat: .2 g (.1 g sat, .1 g mono, 0 g poly)
Protein: .3 g and 4%

Carbohydrate: 6.6 g and 91%
Fiber: .4 g
Cholesterol: 0 mg
Iron: .2 mg

Sodium: 1.3 mg
Calcium: 3.9 mg
Diabetic Exchanges:
½ Other Carbohydrate

# Raspberry Sauce Sweetened with Fruit Juice

*Raspberries' vibrant fresh flavor is preserved in this smooth and bright-red sauce by lightly thickening it with gelatin rather than cooking and thickening with cornstarch or arrowroot. The sweetener is fruit juice concentrate.*

YIELD: 1½ c sauce
SERVING SIZE: 3 tbsp sauce

SERVINGS: 8

| | WEIGHT | MEASURE |
|---|---|---|
| Unflavored gelatin | | ½ tsp |
| Thawed white grape juice concentrate, undiluted | | ½ c + 1 tbsp |
| Fresh ripe raspberries or frozen unsweetened raspberries | 12 oz | 3 c (1½ pt) |
| Almond extract | | ¼ tsp |

Sprinkle gelatin over grape juice concentrate in a small saucepan. Let stand until it swells to a spongy consistency, or about 5 minutes. Place over low heat, stirring until gelatin is completely dissolved. Remove from heat.

Combine raspberries, gelatin mixture, and almond extract in a blender or food processor. Blend until smooth. Strain through a fine mesh strainer (to remove seeds) into a storage container. Ladle over desserts such as Baileys Irish Cream Chocolate Cake (page 61) and serve.

---

### NUTRITIONAL FACTS

| | | |
|---|---|---|
| Calories: 51 (5% from fat) | Carbohydrate: 12 g and 89% | Iron: .3 mg |
| Fat: .3 g (0 g sat, 0 g mono, .2 g poly) | Alcohol: .1 g and 1% | Sodium: 1.4 mg |
| Protein: .6 g and 5% | Fiber: 2.9 g | Calcium: 11.5 mg |
| | Cholesterol: 0 mg | Diabetic Exchanges: 1 Fruit |

# Summer-Fresh Three Berry Sauce

*Ripe berries have a lot going for them. They are one of the sweetest foods (except cranberries), contain few calories, and are full of vitamins, minerals, and fiber. Furthermore, preliminary research reported in the* UC Berkeley Wellness Letter *indicates that berries may be good for our health, too. Studies have found that extracts from all three of the berries in this sauce—strawberries, blueberries, and raspberries—may help protect against various kinds of cancer. So buy enough to make this sauce—and a few extra to snack on.*

YIELD: 2 c (1 pt) sauce and berries    SERVINGS: 8
SERVING SIZE: ¼ c sauce and berries

|  | WEIGHT | MEASURE |
|---|---|---|
| Fresh ripe raspberries, divided | 6 oz | 1⅓ c |
| Fresh ripe blueberries, divided | 6 oz | 1¼ c |
| Fresh ripe hulled strawberries, halved and divided | 6 oz | 1 c |
| Granulated sugar | 1 oz | 2 tbsp |
| Gewurztraminer wine |  | 2 tbsp |
| Fresh lemon juice |  | 1 tbsp |

Combine 3 ounces (half) of each berry and sugar in a small saucepan. Cook over low heat, stirring, until berries begin to cook down and thicken.

Add wine and lemon juice. Simmer, stirring, until wine has reduced and mixture is sauce consistency. Strain through a fine mesh strainer (to remove seeds) into a storage container. Refrigerate until chilled.

Combine remaining berries in a medium bowl. Drizzle sauce and sprinkle berries over desserts such as Lemon-Flavored Cheesecake in Graham Cracker Crumb Crust (page 150) or a scoop of vanilla low-fat ice cream and serve.

## *VARIATION*

Warm Three Berry Sauce: Cook all berries in sauce and serve warm.

## NUTRITIONAL FACTS

Calories: 43 (5% from fat)
Fat: .3 g (0 g sat, 0 g
  mono, .1 g poly)
Protein: .5 g and 4%

Carbohydrate: 10.5 g and
  89%
Alcohol: .1 g and 2%
Fiber: 2.5 g
Cholesterol: 0 mg

Iron: .2 mg
Sodium: 1.6 mg
Calcium: 9.1 mg
Diabetic Exchanges:
  ½ Fruit

# Whipped Light
# Cream Cheese Frosting

*This smooth and creamy fat-free cream cheese frosting, like its higher-fat counterpart, makes a delicious complement to rich and moist fruit and vegetable-based cookies, bars, and cakes such as Old-Fashioned Carrot Pineapple Raisin Cake (page 78), Pumpkin Roulade Rolled with Cream Cheese Frosting (page 81), and Whole Wheat Banana Zucchini Cake Studded with Pineapple and Raisins (page 85).*

YIELD: 1 c frosting
SERVING SIZE: 1 tbsp frosting

SERVINGS: 16

|  | WEIGHT | MEASURE |
|---|---|---|
| Block-style fat-free cream cheese | 6 oz | ¾ c |
| Sifted powdered sugar | 2½ oz | ½ c + 2 tbsp |
| Vanilla extract |  | ½ tsp |

Combine all ingredients in a small mixing bowl. Beat with a mixer until light and creamy. Use as a topping or filling for cakes. Store refrigerated.

## NUTRITIONAL FACTS

Calories: 27 (0% from fat)
Fat: 0 g
Protein: 1.5 g and 24%
Carbohydrate: 4.8 g and
  76%

Fiber: 0 g
Cholesterol: 1.9 mg
Iron: 0 mg
Sodium: 63.7 mg

Calcium: .1 mg
Diabetic Exchanges:
  ½ Other Carbohydrate

# Index

nuts
  nutty chocolate peanut butter brownies,
    102–103
  pecans, toasting, 14
  toasting, 112

oatmeal
  and apple breakfast dessert, baked,
    116–117
  raisin pie with pure maple syrup,
    155–156
oats
  apple crisp with brown sugar oat top-
    ping, 36–37
  blueberry oat bran muffins laced with
    cinnamon, 118–119
  cranberry oat muffins with a hint of
    orange, 122–123
  hot peach tart on oat bran crust, 148–149
  nutrition in, 116, 155
  purple plum blueberry oat crunch,
    51–52
  rolled, 122
  wholesome apple spice oat bars, 109–110
  whole wheat oat muffins speckled with
    dried cherries, 135–136
oils, 4–5, 112
oranges
  apricot soy bread flavored with orange,
    113–114
  baked pear halves stuffed with dates in
    aromatic orange syrup, 40–41
  cranberry oat muffins with a hint of
    orange, 122–123
  cranberry white whole wheat bread
    flavored with orange, 124–125
  layered raspberries, Bing cherries, and,
    23–24
  lemon sauce dancing with lemon, lime,
    and orange zests, 222–223
  navel, and kiwis sprinkled with berries
    in rose-scented syrup, 26–27
  orange fat-free and sugar-free sherbet,
    191–192
  orange-flavored meringue pastry shell,
    175

orange marshmallow meringue topping,
    172
orange powdered sugar frosting with
    finely grated zest, 224
orange sections in raspberry syrup
    splashed with Chambord, 27–28
pumpkin chiffon pie dashed with
    orange in corn flake crumb crust,
    159–160
rhubarb strawberry pie with a hint of
    orange and cinnamon, 162–163
sectioning, 18

pancakes, whole wheat
  gingerbread, 134–135
  strawberry, studded with strawberry
    bits, 137–138
pandowdy, defined, 48
papaya
  banana sauce sweetened with fruit
    juice, 28–29
  ripening of, 28
parfaits, fresh fruit, peach yogurt, and
    granola, 20
peaches
  baked banana peach crumble with
    gingersnap topping, 38–39
  creamy banana and peach sherbet,
    185–187
  fresh fruit, peach yogurt, and granola
    parfaits, 20
  fuzz on commercially grown, 211
  hot peach tart on oat bran crust,
    148–149
  and just-like-cream smoothie, 211
  meringue-topped blueberry stuffed
    poached peach halves, 47–48
  peach and strawberry frozen yogurt,
    192–194
  peach blackberry crumble with whole
    wheat topping, 48–49
  peach pie topped with lemon marshmal-
    low meringue, 156–157
  removing skin from, 32, 47
  rum-flavored sour cream gelatin dotted
    with, 54–55